SHOULDER PAIN?

THE SOLUTION & PREVENTION

Fir ... ON
Revised & Expanded

BY

JOHN M. KIRSCH, M.D.

THE KIRSCH INSTITUTE FOR SHOULDER RESEARCH LLC
IN ASSOCIATION WITH BOOKSTAND PUBLISHING

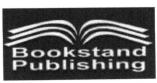

www.kirschshoulder.com   www.bookstandpublishing.com

Published by
The Kirsch Institute for Shoulder Research LLC
In Association with Bookstand Publishing
3056_24

ISBN 978-1-58909-642-4

First Edition: January 2010
Second Edition: February 2011
Third Edition: March 2012
Fourth Edition: January 2013
Fifth Edition: July 2019

"Let us affirm what seems to be the truth..."

– Plato, *"The Republic,"* Bk. VIII

"Science is about defining truths about nature, through experiment, or; <u>experience</u>."

– Richard Feynman (nuclear physicist)

My purpose in writing this book for the public is to *empower* you to restore and maintain the health of your own shoulders and help you avoid unnecessary therapy and surgery. This sense of *empowerment* will allow you to control your own exercise program without the reflex resistance that occurs when another person attempts to stretch your shoulder or direct your exercise program.

In addition, I bring to your attention the large number of shoulder surgeries performed that provide no benefit and that carry risks of serious complications and harm. For example, studies have shown that the most common shoulder surgery, subacromial decompression (SAD) with its exorbitant cost and complications is no more effective than a guided exercise program. This is discussed further in the book. As you read through this book be mindful that the information in the book is the opinion of one orthopedic surgeon. You may prefer to take the counsel of your own physician.

The exercises in the book are simple.

The research for the book was not.

CONTENTS

Acknowledgements viii

Introduction ix

Preface xiii

The CA Arch xv

Six Aspects xvi

The Kauai Study xvii

Osteoarthritis xix

Gravity is Free! xxi

A Word About Inversion Hanging xxii

The Computer Tomography (CT) Scan Technique for Simulating
   the Hanging Position xxiii

Some Edited CT Scan Images After Scanning xxv

Raw Images Captured with the CT Scanner Before Editing xxviii

Testimonials xxxii

Part One: The Enigma of the Shoulder

My Story: Solving the Enigma of the Shoulder 3

As the Twig is Bent: How the Shoulder is Remodeled by Hanging 9

Beginnings of Shoulder Problems 11

A Little Shoulder Anatomy 12

The New Joint in the Shoulder, The Acromiohumeral Joint 13

Usual Presentation of Shoulder Anatomy 15

The Skeleton Seen While Hanging 16

The Scapulothoracic Joint 17

Shoulder Muscles and Tendons 18

Acromial Shapes 19

Cadaver Shoulder View..20

CT Scan Images While Hanging 21

Acromiohumeral Joint Close-up View 22

The Exercises...23

The Hanging Exercise 26

People Hanging...28

Partial/Reduced Weight Hanging 31

Lifting Weights...33

Model Lifting Weights 35

The Most Common Shoulder Problems 38

The Subacromial Impingement Syndrome (SIS)....................39

Relieving the Impingement by Hanging 40

The Subacromial Decompression Surgery (SAD)..................44

The Kirsch Institute Theory: The Hanging Exercise Relieves the
Subacromial Impingement Syndrome/Subacromial Pain
Syndrome Without Surgery 45

The Torn Rotator Cuff..46

The Frozen Shoulder (Adhesive Capsulitis)............................48

Some Suggestions for Hanging Equipment 50

Part Two: The Science

The Coracoacromial (CA) Arch...57

Another Joint in the Shoulder: The Acromiohumeral Joint 61

Close-up View..63

The Acromiohumeral Joint: X-ray View 64

The Two Main Joints in the Shoulder 66

The Acromiohumeral Interval: X-ray View.............................67

CT Scan View of the Shoulder in a Simulated Hanging Position 69

Slice or Axial Images..70

The Subacromial Bursa..72
Subacromial Decompression Surgery 74
Shoulder CT Scan: Front View 77
Bending the Acromion by Hanging..78
Arm Elevation Versus Hanging..79
The Acromiohumeral Joint: CT Scan Views 82
Finding the CAL...84
The Humerus Bends the Acromion While Hanging...........86
The Human Pendulum 87
Muscles Stretched While Hanging...89
Hanging for the Spine..90
The Importance of Hanging Through the Ages 91

Epilogue...93
Bibliography...97

Acknowledgements

With gratitude to my wife Joy for her encouragement and belief in the importance of this book and to my daughter Lorelei for acting as the model; and to all who have validated the exercise program in the book by restoring the health of their own shoulders.

Introduction

This book is about an exercise that heals the shoulder and a new joint in the human body, the "acromiohumeral" joint. Because of the importance of discovering this joint I have repeated images of the joint many times throughout the book.

It is by engaging this joint by hanging from an overhead bar that the shoulder is healed and maintained. The rest of the book is my explanation of why and how it works. At first, the exercise may seem counter-intuitive because it is painful. After time, the pain subsides and is replaced with a feeling of well-being.

The hanging exercise is not a panacea! The hanging exercise is not recommended for persons with unstable or dislocating shoulders, in precarious physical health, or with severe osteoporosis (fragile bones). If you have shoulder pain that goes unexplained for several weeks it is wise to obtain a diagnosis from your physician.

It's been five years since I wrote the Fourth Edition. Taking the advice of family, friends and critics, I decided it was time to update the book. I have added many testimonials/reviews, as well as some additional helpful images. I have also updated the website: www.kirschshoulder.com. Although it is not necessary for the reader to study or understand the images in the book to benefit from the exercises, I believe that most will benefit from viewing them.

In writing this book for the public and medical professionals, I have tried my best to keep the vocabulary to the common English language. In spite of this, I found it necessary to use the scientific Latin terms where necessary.

I wrote this book to provide an exercise program that restores and maintains the health of the shoulder without the need for pills, therapy or surgery. When I realized that I could help people avoid unnecessary surgery, the writing and publication of the book became a moral obligation. When I graduated from medical school I took the Hippocratic Oath, which states in part:

"To consider dear to me, as my parents, him who taught me this art; to live in common with him and, if necessary share my goods with him; to look upon his children as my own brothers, to teach them this art; and that by my teaching, I will impart a knowledge of this art to my own sons, and to my teacher's sons, and to disciples bound by an indenture and oath according to the medical laws, and no other. I will prescribe regimens for the good of my patients according to my ability and my judgment and never do harm to anyone."

In 2004 I wrote an academic paper on the shoulder and submitted it for publication. Then months later, finding that it wouldn't be published, it became a moral imperative to write this book for the public. I had access to a computer tomography (CT) scanner and a program that allowed me to capture, edit and save the CT scan images that are in the book. I already knew that hanging from a bar healed my shoulders but I didn't know why. My purpose in making the CT scans then was to learn what happens to the shoulder anatomy when a person hangs from a bar so that I could then impart this knowledge to the public. After studying these images, I realized I had discovered a new joint in the shoulder, the acromiohumeral joint. This joint has never been previously discovered, imaged or explained. It is by engaging this joint doing the hanging exercise that you restore and maintain the health of your shoulders. I have included the

CT scan images of this joint in the book to allow you to visualize what is happening while you're doing the exercises that remodel your shoulders. These scans present the shoulder anatomy in 3D images and videos and will greatly enhance your understanding of shoulder anatomy and the hanging exercise. Without these images the rationale for the exercise program would be mere speculation. With the CT images the hanging exercise is validated. These images have unlocked the mystery of shoulder biomechanics. Videos of these images are available on the website www.kirschshoulder.com and at YouTube under "Dr. John Kirsch."

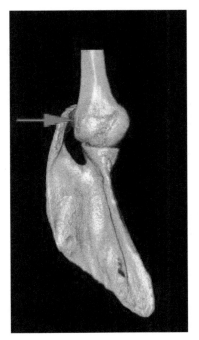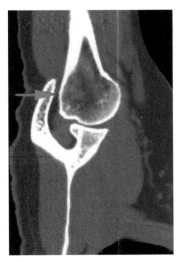

Fig. 1 These two images show the acromiohumeral joint (red arrows), the new joint in the shoulder that is visible when doing the simulated hanging exercise in a CT scanner (explained on page xxiii).

This joint, the acromiohumeral joint, allows you to heal and maintain your shoulders by hanging from a bar. The humerus leans on and bends the acromion (explained throughout the book).

Many ask why, instead of publishing the information in a scientific journal, I wrote this book for the public. If I had done the former, the information in the book would molder in libraries for many years instead of reaching the people who need it now; those with shoulder pain.

After I wrote the Fourth Edition I had hoped orthopedic surgeons would somehow find the book and consider giving their patients the option of trying the exercises in the book before resorting to surgery. Some physical therapists, trainers and chiropractors have found the book by word of mouth or online and are using the exercises with good success for their patients and athletes. In light of the excellent results from the exercise program for the past eight years, it is a mystery to me why physicians have not acknowledged or adopted the exercise program for their patients.

An old Latin proverb, *"Repetitio est Mater Studiorum,"* or *"Repetition is the Mother of Study,"* tells us that to learn, we must repeat. Following this rule, I have repeated some of the information and images in the book.

There are many photos and descriptions of shoulder anatomy in the book that might seem formidable for many. But as you read through the book I believe you will find that this material is not that difficult to grasp. I have tried my best to simplify and explain the otherwise complicated anatomy.

Preface

The model pictured in Fig. 2 on the next page and on the cover is hanging from an overhead bar. This is the exercise that will remodel your shoulders, relieve the subacromial impingement syndrome, the frozen shoulder and prevent pinching and tearing the rotator cuff as well as relieve back pain by decompressing the disc spaces. Along with simple weight lifting, the exercise will maintain the health of your shoulders and in most cases make pills, therapy and surgery unnecessary. Not all will be able to do the full hanging exercise. Some will initially need to do partial or limited weight hanging keeping their feet on a stool or floor. This is further explained later on page 31.

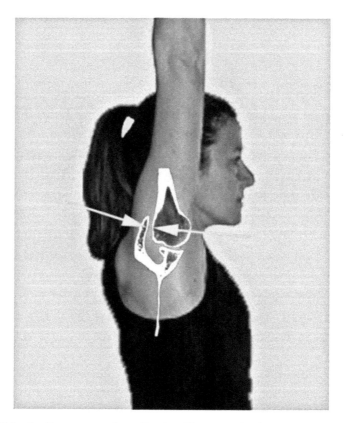

Fig. 2 This is the exercise that will stretch the arch of ligament and bone, the coracoacromial arch, the CA arch (see **Figs. 3** and **68**), which may cause shoulder pain and rotator cuff injury if not stretched. A CT scan slice image of a shoulder made in the simulated hanging position is over-laid on the model's shoulder to depict the biomechanics of the exercise. In this figure, notice how the humerus is positioned to lean against the acromion part of the scapula (yellow arrows, acromion on the left, humerus on the right). The space between the yellow arrows is the new joint in the shoulder, the acromiohumeral joint. It is the pressure applied to the acromion by the humerus while hanging that maintains the health of the shoulder. The evidence shows that hanging from a bar relieves the symptoms of the subacromial impingement syndrome, rotator cuff injury and the frozen shoulder.

The Coracoacromial Arch
(the CA Arch)

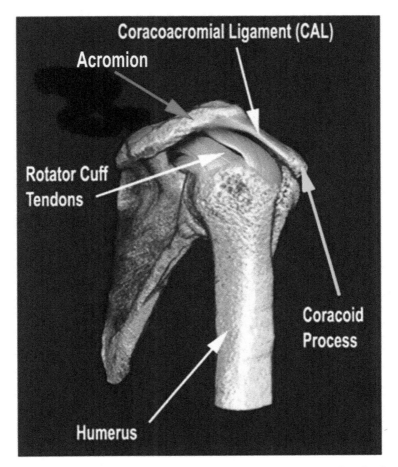

Fig. 3 It is essential to understand the CA arch. It is this structure that becomes deformed with time, gravity, and neglect, and then presses on the structures below, causing damage to the rotator cuff and subacromial bursa. This is discussed throughout the book. The CA arch: red arrow: acromion, white arrow: the coracoacromial ligament, green arrow: the coracoid process.

Six Aspects

1. **Fact:** Hanging from a bar and lifting light weights relieves most shoulder pain problems.

2. **The Exercise Program:** Hanging from an overhead bar and lifting light weights.

3. **Theory:** My theory as to why the exercise program works to relieve shoulder pain.

4. **Explains** a never before mentioned joint in the shoulder, the acromiohumeral joint, and why engaging this joint by hanging heals and prevents injury to the shoulder. This is explained in detail throughout the book.

5. **Redundancy:** There is a redundancy in the human body that allows other structures to take over when one is lost. Other muscles can take over when the rotator cuff is torn. Nature supplies us with back-ups.

6. **Relieving back pain:** Hanging is the only exercise that can safely stretch the spine imparting a distraction force to decompress the disc spaces and relieve back pain.

The Kauai Study

In March 2012 I presented the first academic study of my research at the 1st Combined Australian/American meeting of the hand and upper extremity societies in Kauai, HI.

The study included 92 carefully followed subjects with shoulder pain problems who used the Kirsch Institute for Shoulder Research exercise program to overcome their shoulder pain.

Many of these subjects had been suffering with shoulder pain for years and had tried other methods of treatment at great expense with no relief. Many were scheduled for, or advised to have shoulder surgery.

The subjects in the study had the following diagnoses:

- **Subacromial Impingement Syndrome (SIS):**   **70**
- **Rotator Cuff (RC) Tears with MRI Diagnosis:**   **16**
- **Adhesive Capsulitis (Frozen Shoulder):**   **4**
- **Osteoarthritis of the Glenohumeral (GH) Joint:**   **2**

Of these 92 subjects, 90 were returned to comfortable ADL (activities of daily living) and remained so after variable years of follow up (1–28 years). Two subjects with shoulder pain had been scheduled to have shoulder replacement surgery and were able to cancel that surgery. Two subjects quit the study for personal reasons.

One person, a 70-year-old woman with osteoarthritis of the GH joint, deserves special mention. She was scheduled for shoulder replacement. I performed a shoulder exam and reviewed her pre-op shoulder x-ray that is shown on the next page.

In light of the excellent success of those following the exercise program in the book, I am no longer recording case studies. I am still writing to readers having questions about their shoulder pain problems at kirschinstitute@gmail.com.

Osteoarthritis

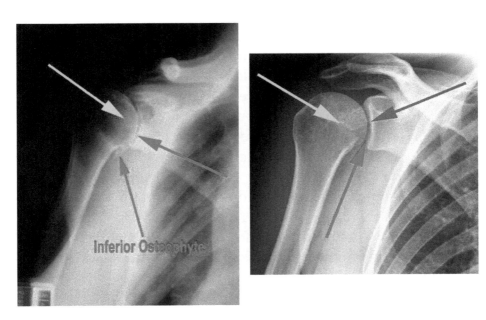

Fig. 4   **Fig 5**

Fig. 4 and **Fig. 5** are X-ray images. In **Fig. 4** The 70-year-old woman subject. Note the narrowed joint space and loss of glenohumeral (GH) joint cartilage, blue arrow; inferior osteophyte (spur), red arrow, humerus, green arrow. Compare this image to **Fig. 5** on the right, a normal shoulder. The glenohumeral (GH) joint with normal cartilage space: red arrow, the humerus, green arrow, and the normal glenoid cavity surface, blue arrow.

This subject had osteoarthritis of the glenohumeral (GH) joint. The cause of her pain was not the arthritis, but severe subacromial impingement syndrome (SIS) and weakness of the rotator cuff (RC) tendons and muscles. She began hanging and weight lifting, cancelled her shoulder replacement surgery and one year later was completely pain-free and returned to cross-country skiing. She continued to improve and could once again shift a standard transmission car. She observed, "little things mean a lot, but not having surgery is a big thing."

That this patient responded to the hanging exercise in spite of the presence of osteoarthritis of the glenohumeral joint presents a new challenge for those surgeons who perform shoulder replacement surgery. The shoulder is not a weight bearing joint as is the hip. For the hip, there is really no other option than joint replacement. But in the case of the shoulder, a person using gravity by hanging can reverse the effects of gravity and relieve their shoulder pain. Not all patients with osteoarthritis of the shoulder have pain from the arthritis, but suffer from subacromial impingement syndrome or rotator cuff disease. That this one patient solved her problem by using the hanging exercise shows us that surgery for osteoarthritis of the shoulder could be delayed until the patient has had the opportunity to attempt relieving the problem with the exercises.

It is my hope that in time, physicians and therapists who treat patients with shoulder pain caused by subacromial impingement (SIS), rotator cuff (RC) tears, frozen shoulder (adhesive capsulitis) and osteoarthritis of the glenohumeral (GH) joint understand and recommend the hanging and weight lifting program outlined in this book before resorting to more invasive procedures.

Gravity is Free!

Or is gravity really free? No, gravity is a blessing and a curse. But it comes at a price. Our anatomy is subject to the force of gravity our entire lives. It pulls us downward keeping us firmly planted on the earth, but at the same time applies a destructive force to our hips, knees, spine and shoulders. There is not much we can do to escape this force. We can minimize the damage to our hips and knees, by maintaining ideal body weight; but to overcome the damage to our shoulders we have another alternative: hanging from an overhead support or bar. When we hang, or brachiate, we reverse the destructive force of gravity and paradoxically use gravity to restore the health of the shoulders. As you will see in the following pages, many elements of the shoulder are stretched to their limit when hanging: a normal human activity.

A Word About Inversion Hanging

People have been hanging in an inverted position (upside-down) since 3000 BC. Hippocrates, the father of medicine recommended inverted hanging in 400BC. Since then many others have recommended the exercise with little evidence that it produces any lasting benefit. Numerous manufacturers have promoted using their inversion machines. The industry has blossomed right up to the present. There may be some serious risks involved with inversion hanging and it should be avoided by those not in the best of health. Hanging from a bar by your hands involves no health risks, restores the health of the shoulders and decompresses the spine.

The Computer Tomography (CT) Scan Technique for Simulating the Hanging Position

For the purpose of understanding why the hanging exercise is so effective, I made CT scans of the shoulder of live subjects, some in a simulated hanging position as well as others in various degrees of arm elevation. These studies present the shoulder both in skeletal and soft tissue formats. The CT scan format allows a far more accurate study of the living body than cadaver studies as the anatomy remains intact and is indeed, "live." Study of the 3D videos will enhance your understanding of the shoulder anatomy and the dynamics of the hanging exercise. I've made some of the videos and still images available on the website: www.kirschshoulder.com

The hanging position is simulated as it is not possible to make CT (computer tomography) scans in the upright hanging position. The scans were created by having the subject hold a 60-pound weight with the arm fully elevated while lying supine on the CT scanner table. Using computer analysis and editing software I captured, edited and saved the images. Viewing these images should allow you to understand how the hanging exercise restores and maintains the health of your shoulders. There is no other research that has studied the shoulder in a hanging position as in this book. This was the first time the shoulder has been x-rayed or scanned in a hanging position. The was the first time the acromiohumeral joint was discovered. You will not find images of the shoulder in a hanging position anywhere else.

I believe the average reader should be able to understand the anatomy as presented. The skeletal images are straight forward.

The "slice" or "axial" images may be a little confusing at first, but with some study should be understandable. The slice image is no different from cutting a branch from a tree and counting the rings. That would be "the anatomy" of a tree, or a "slice" of a tree seen on end or cross-section (see **Fig. 78**).

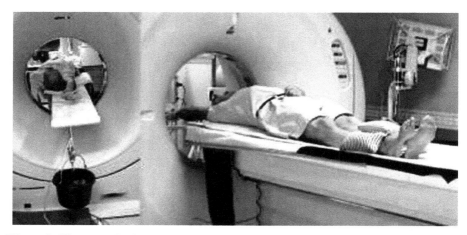

Fig. 6 The technique used to simulate the overhead hanging position. The subject lies supine on the CT scanner table holding a rope attached to a bucket holding a 60lb weight. The 60lb weight approximates the force on the shoulder while hanging from an overhead bar. The supine posture is the only position possible with current CT scanners. This position does allow a close simulation of the anatomy in the vertical hanging position. The CT scan takes only 45 seconds whereas an MRI would take 45 minutes; it would be very difficult for a subject to hold the weight for that long.

Some Edited CT Scan Images After Scanning

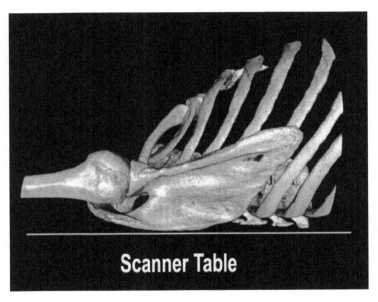

Fig. 7 Shoulder and ribs lying supine simulating hanging after limited editing. This image shows the shoulder and chest skeleton while lying in the scanner holding a 60lb weight.

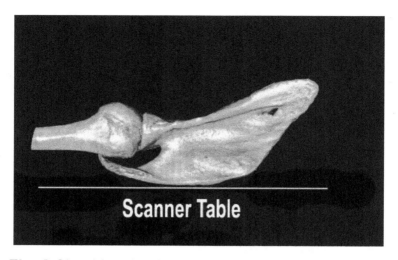

Fig. 8 Shoulder simulating hanging with further editing.

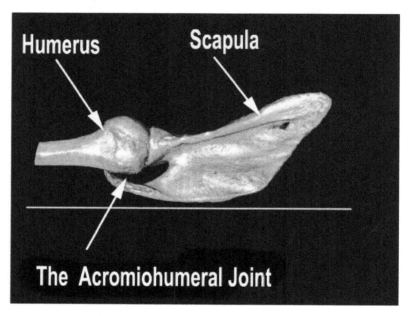

Fig. 9 Shoulder in scanner showing the new joint in the shoulder, the "acromiohumeral joint."

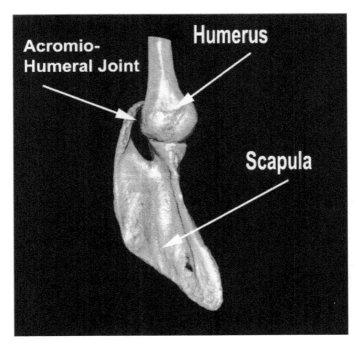

Fig. 10 Following the CT scan, the shoulder has this appearance when hanging.

Raw Images Captured with the CT Scanner Before Editing

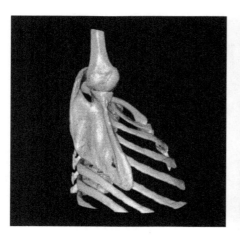

Fig. 11

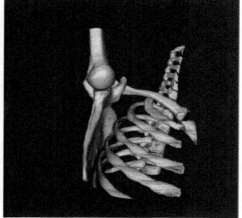

Fig. 12

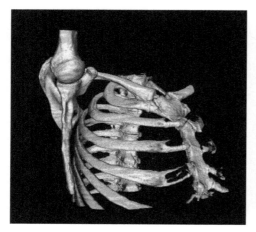

Fig. 13

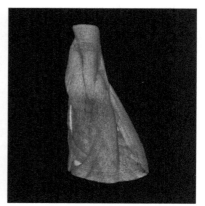

Fig. 14

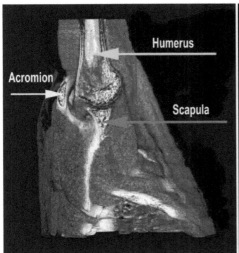
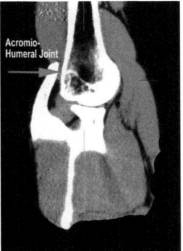

Fig. 15   **Fig. 16**

These figures demonstrate the type of images captured with the CT scanner before editing. They show the shoulder structures while simulating hanging from a bar.

Following the CT scan, the image files were then downloaded, studied and edited saving the images that best explain the anatomy of the shoulder in a hanging position. **In Fig. 15** a soft tissue CT image while simulating hanging. In **Fig. 16** the acromiohumeral joint, the new joint in the shoulder (red arrow).

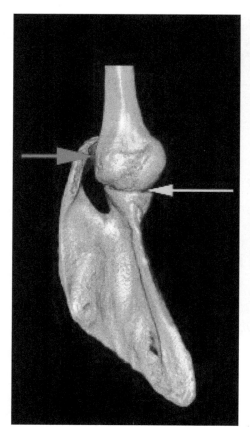
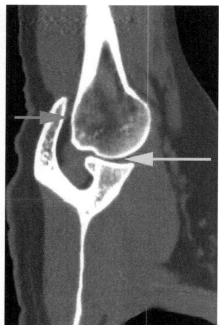

Fig. 17   Fig. 18

Shoulder CT scans taken in a simulated hanging position after editing. **Fig. 17**, 3D view, **Fig. 18**, saggital slice view. These images are explained and repeated as you read through the book. Red arrows: the acromiohumeral joint. Green arrows: the glenohumeral joint.

Throughout the book you will find that I have deliberately repeated some of the images to emphasize their importance in helping you understand how the exercises in the book solve shoulder pain problems. It is wisely said that *"one picture is worth a thousand words."*

I have found that failure to exercise the acromiohumeral joint is the leading cause of shoulder pain in the adult. My research has shown that relief of this pain can almost always be obtained with a simple exercise program and almost never requires surgical intervention. The findings of a rotator cuff tear are almost always attritional (wearing away) and age related.

Testimonials

Testimonials/book reviews are stories told by persons relating their experiences. Readers have commented that they wished there were more testimonials/reviews in the book, so I have added these for this edition. Reading the experiences of persons who used the exercises in the book to relieve their shoulder pain is probably the best way to appreciate the power of the exercise program. These testimonials are mostly taken from Amazon book reviews. Many have contacted me personally at kirschinstitute@gmail.com relating their enthusiasm for the exercise program that solved their shoulder problems in days, weeks or months without pills, therapy or surgery. The many readers relating their success with the exercise program, more than any other evidence validates the program. I hope that by reading these stories you will be encouraged to persevere with the exercise program.

These testimonials might be considered "anecdotal" evidence and be disregarded by some as "unscientific." The testimonial is an observation made by an individual with the experience. Anecdotal evidence can be within the scope of the scientific method and be both empirical and verifiable. If a doctor confirms the observation, it is called a clinical case study, and therefore acceptable as medical evidence. The many people using the exercises in the book who have solved their shoulder pain problems without pills, therapy or surgery constitutes a large population of successful medical case studies that then becomes useful medical evidence.

So here are some stories that show how the exercises have worked to relieve most shoulder pain problems:

2019 SB Dear Dr. Kirsch,

Thank you so much for your amazing book and research on shoulder pain. I have begun using your hanging technique with great success in my physical therapy practice.

* * * * *

2018 Rob S. in the UK

"Absolutely amazing!"

"I am 77. I had a torn rotator cuff, severe arthritis, impingement, virtually everything that can be wrong with the shoulder. Saw a surgeon who said there was so much going on in my shoulder he decided not to operate because even if he repaired the cuff, it was likely to tear again. It got steadily worse; couldn't raise the arm above the horizontal, could not sleep on that side, could not use the computer mouse etc., etc. In desperation I bought this book and religiously followed its advice. Be warned, the initial pain of hanging is out of this world - but must be endured! Absolutely amazing! I am totally cured! Within just a couple of sessions I could even sleep on the affected side. The shoulder is a bit noisy, but NO pain now at all. Back in the gym, and doing exercises I'd been unable to do for years. As strong as the other shoulder.

God bless Dr Kirsch. If the rotator cuff is still torn, it's not bothering me. Dr Kirsch says other structures take over. They certainly have in my case. I hang for a minimum of two 35 second sessions a day. Regarding the reviewer who complains that the book is about just one thing, hanging from a bar; why on earth does that matter if the method works??? It DOES work! Absolutely amazing, a total and almost instant cure to a very severe problem."

* * * * *

2018 PDX123 "Very quickly got me back to the kind of life I thought I'd lost forever."

"One-year update: still a freaking miracle; and this old lady will arm wrestle all naysayers! If you aren't already hanging, but are taking time to read this review, just buy the book. I honestly don't hang every day, still don't have a real bar, but occasional hanging has kept my shoulders fully functioning and pain free for a year now. Really feels good for my back, too, when it gets sore from all the heavy lifting I do.

6-month review:

Total miracle for a nonbeliever! The book looks hokey, but buy it. Knowing how well it works, this was worth a fortune to me. It was other reviewers here and on YouTube that convinced me to try this after 10 months of pain and life limitations from torn rotator cuff and severely frozen shoulder, so I'll add my testimony as a former skeptic.

Yes, a one-word synopsis is accurate: HANG. If you're reading this review and haven't already reshaped your shoulders by hanging, then buy the dang book, read it, criticize it in your mind, google Dr. Kirsch and wonder if he's still alive and why his website is so funky, THEN HANG! Then bless his name as your shoulder savior forever. The book does show the way hanging reshapes your shoulder anatomy and I needed to see that as a skeptic who was too scared/lazy/dumb to just try hanging without the book.

I was ready to spend tens of thousands on iffy surgery just to be able to live with the pain. I was a middle-aged woman with one shoulder about ten years post rotator cuff tear and the other one badly torn ten months before and completely and painfully frozen for many of those months. I just wanted to be able to sleep through the night, maybe brush my hair, and had totally given up hope of ever getting back to the sports and activities of my younger years. I was considering manipulation under anesthesia, read a lot of publications on the high instance of broken bones, low instance of happy shoulders one, two, five, ten years later and was very discouraged.

Basically, I could not imagine how my arm could get up to a hanging position ever again, but saw with manipulation they just yank it up there under anesthesia. Sometimes it breaks the arm, but I figured I was ready to pay someone a fortune to drug me, give a quick yank to tear through all the scar-like encapsulating "frozen" tissue, maybe break my arm, very likely leave me back with the same problem or even worse soon after, then I could try to do it myself with a more incremental approach.

I was honestly scared to try to hang, as it hurt to barely jostle my arm. I especially worried for too long how exactly, I should move all the way from the barely 45 degrees I could push my arm to somehow hanging with my hands overhead. To even get my upper arm parallel with the floor I had to use the other hand to push it and had to cheat with extreme contortion of my torso and hunching. The detail of how exactly to "hang" from there isn't really explained in the book, but I'll tell you how awkwardly I started what seemed impossible.

So, try it like I finally did. With bent elbows down, and hands up, I finally just grabbed what I could reach-the top of my shower tub's door frame. The "bar" was only a few inches higher than my shoulders, about eye level. Once I had grabbed it, I bent my knees just a little to drop my body down a bit and leaned back just a little.

So, I tried the fake hanging again a little later in the day and a few times the next day. By the third day my horribly frozen shoulder was unbelievably unfreezing. By the third week, I was thrilled to be working out. Internal and external rotating with strong therapy bands, lifting 8lb dumbbells overhead, etc.

I honestly did not put a lot of effort into this, but it was enough to quickly transform my shoulders (and my life). I like adrenaline sports and hate gyms and boring working out stuff. I still don't hang my full body weight because I've been too lazy to put up a bar. Most days, once or twice a day, I grab the top of a door frame, a metal cabinet at work, or my shower door and only sort of bent-knee hang, but I can now relax into it, feel my shoulders rotate normally up around my ears, and open up the joint as that arch thing gets bent. At any hint of shoulder pain, stiffness or impinging, I'll look for something I can sort of hang from - a metal cabinet at work, stair railings in my parking garage, or whatever I can use to stretch that arm out and open up the shoulder. I do just a few exercises with therapy bands over a door and dumbbells, and both my shoulders are now fully ripped after a decade of being torn and/or frozen.

Now, six months later, I can't believe it, I can do anything I was doing two decades ago. I had torn my other rotator cuff about ten years ago. I was told it would never heal on its own, but I procrastinated on surgery and it maybe 70% healed over three years. I still can't reach very high behind my back, but who cares? I'm a 50yr old woman, working on cars over my head, windsurfing, kayaking, and now I think I'll try kiteboarding."

* * * * *

2019 RS "I appreciate receiving your book. Since February, I have applied the technique outlined in the book. I was barely able to even lift my arm at the time. Now full range with no limitation. Thank you.

2017 James T.

*"For years, I had shoulder problems. Then, a few years ago I found this book. Its revolutionary approach fixed my shoulders for good. I'm 70, and my shoulders feel loose, strong, and free. If you have Frozen Shoulder DO NOT THINK, just buy it. Buy this book! It is a gem. Six years ago I had a frozen shoulder. It will usually go away by itself after 30 months, but you have to suffer the pain and the uncomfortable sleep and not be able to use your arm for everyday errands, I used pain killers with heat and ice and ultrasound treatments and acupuncture and it went away after 3 months. And then the frozen shoulder came back without any reason like the last time, and I suffered with the pain for almost 2 months until I read this book. STILL I do not believe how fast it took away the pain and the limited range of movement in just 8 days (**8 DAYS**). The book price should be 100 times the actual price because you will be cured fast and will not pay doctors anything; do not think anymore, BUY and read this book."*

* * * * *

2017 Sojourner More than worth every penny!

This method really helps! I had a very stiff right arm that had lost a lot of range of motion. I bought this book and a hanging bar that I could put up in a doorway in my house and now six months later I have full use of my arms again. No drugs, no paid therapy etc. Very happy I found this method!

* * * * *

2017 Dori O'Rourke "It's not your age!"

"It was the last day of the 2017 basketball tournament when I noticed something was going on in my right shoulder. When I got back home, I started doing traditional shoulder rehabilitation exercises, but gradually my shoulder kept getting worse and worse. A month after Nationals, I couldn't even lift my arm without pain.

Everyone was telling me how hard shoulders were to heal and that it would take months. I was starting to believe they might be right when I discovered some videos on YouTube that made perfect sense to me and my sports medicine brain. The videos were about a simple thing we could all do to heal our shoulders. It was being touted by an Orthopedic Surgeon named Dr. John Kirsch. I followed the simple shoulder protocol and was very happily surprised at how fast the pain subsided and how quickly I was able to get back on the basketball court and play again. Because of the great results I had, since that time if I ever hear about anyone who's having shoulder issues, I send them those videos. All my friends, family, golf students and basketball buddies who have followed the videos have had similar success. If you're dealing with impingement or a rotator cuff issue, I highly recommend that you start doing what Dr. Kirsch recommends."

Dori O'Rourke

Co-Founder/CEO, SPORTS after 50.org
30+ Year LPGA Teaching Professional
Movement Restoration Specialist
SPORTSafter50.org
Author, "It's NOT your AGE!"

* * * * *

2019 Amazon Customer "Absolute Life Saver"

"Background: I had a full thickness rotator cuff tear from a snowboarding fall. At the time I was 25 y/o. An orthopedist laughed at me when I asked if I could fix the pain with physical therapy. He insisted surgery was my only route. I have nothing against the doc or any doc, but he said the sole way to fix the pain would be to get the surgery. I had already spent hundreds of hours researching how I could fix my torn rotator cuff when I had finally given up and scheduled the DREADED surgery.

It wasn't until 2 days before the surgery that I found this book and decided to cancel or postpone the surgery for one last shot to heal myself after reading all these positive reviews. It WORKS.

It's been about a year now since I started hanging (I stopped maybe 3 months in). Though I will never forget the pain, the popping and crackling sounds of my first hang, it was well worth it. I went from being barely able to lift my hand above my head to today having no issues. It wasn't until I had stopped hanging that my shoulder was completely healed.

I used to not be able to even sleep on my side and now I'm back to my normal activities like weight lifting, golfing and snow-boarding. If you were anything like me where I was depressed and angry that I couldn't physically do the activities that I loved anymore. BUY THIS BOOK AND Try IT!"

2012 Richard S. "If you have shoulder pain, get this!"

"Sometime over a year ago, my right shoulder began to hurt a lot, and I lost a lot of range of motion with my right arm. Typically, I ignore such problems, and eventually they go away. Last summer, I realized it wasn't going away. Instead, the pain was waking me up in the middle of the night. I couldn't sleep on my right side. I couldn't grab high things with my right hand. Finally, I was forced to acknowledge I had a problem, so I began researching it online, and finally concluded I must have some degree of torn rotator cuff, perhaps from sleeping on that side or perhaps from doing too many pushups. I tried other books and their shoulder exercises helped relieve the pain temporarily, but were no solution.

Finally, I found this one, and I'm grateful. It's a short book, and much of the material consists of testimonials. The actual technique consists of doing two things, one essential and the other supportive of the first. Fortunately, I was able to find a playground in my neighborhood with a swing set with a bar I could use, and I began hanging nearly every day. The first time it was some of the worst pain I'd ever felt. Prepare to hurt a lot at first. But don't stop. The more I did it, the less pain I felt during that period, and certainly the less pain I felt for the remainder of the day and night. Now I'm practically pain free. I still have some motion limits, which I believe is because I no longer hang regularly."

2018 E.A. "Able to avoid surgery and to return to full function"

"I found the book to be very engaging, practical and clinically scientific. The CT scans were very convincing in showing the effectiveness of the methods. I had damage to my right rotator cuff and stiffness in the left. I have been using the stretching and exercises for about 5 months and progress has been steady and successful. I have full range of motion in both shoulders and very little discomfort anymore. Plan to continue regimen as daily routine to prevent further issues. I am 73 and hope to get stronger with time."

2019 Paul K. "Great Book"

"This treatment works very well, it's easy and free. No need for rotator cuff surgery! Nice CT scan pictures for skeptical therapists and doctors."

* * * * *

2012 Rick Newcombe, Creators Syndicate, Hermosa Beach, California

"I highly recommend this book...to Everyone, those with shoulder pain and everyone else-because Dr. Kirsch's hanging exercises and light dumbbell exercises will heal most shoulder ailments and prevent future episodes from occurring.

My first encounter with shoulder pain occurred when I was 50. It was my right shoulder, and the pain was very severe, forcing me to use light weights. I did a ton of high-rep shoulder exercises using 2- and 3-pound dumbbells. The pain finally subsided after three months. Then, five years later, the pain came back with a vengeance.

I saw an orthopedic surgeon, who said, after a series of tests, that I had a rotator cuff tear and was a candidate for shoulder surgery. I would get cortisone shots and feel relief for a few days, and then the pain would return. As I was considering surgery, I started reading everything I could find on shoulder injuries. I read dozens of books and hundreds of articles and then, at some point with all this reading, I discovered an earlier edition of the book you have in your hands, and my life was changed. Once I found Dr. Kirsch's book, I ordered it for my Kindle. Once I started reading it, I couldn't put it down. What I loved about Dr. Kirsch's approach was that he was saying it was up to me to heal my shoulder; not some passive solution like lying unconscious on a hospital bed while a surgeon chipped away at my shoulder bone to create more room This was incredible-that my treatment was up to me, that I could remodel my shoulder through my own hard work, as opposed to a passive solution such as having a surgeon cut into the bone, or massage therapy or any of the other passive solutions for shoulder therapy. I then bought the paperback version of the book to be able to study the pictures better.

Dr. Kirsch said that by regular hanging I could create the room between bones myself. Initially I found it difficult to hang with full body weight for more than 10 sec. At some point, 10 seconds became 20 and then eventually 30, which meant that I could hang from a bar

comfortably for 30 sec. Well, that is what I did, and now, one year later, I hang at least six days a week for a minimum of 30 seconds doing 30 reps in each of those sets.

Sometimes I will hang for a full minute, just to test myself. I don't mind the calluses on my hands, but if you do, you can always wear weight lifting gloves. I have seen that my body actually gets taller during a hang, where if I start with my feet three inches off the ground, by the end of 30 seconds my shoes are practically standing flat while I hang. I am not saying that hanging will make you taller, but I suspect it will help in slowing down the natural shrinking of the spine that comes with old age. This treatment has been life changing because I feel young again. Well, that is what I did, and now, one year later, I hang at least six days a week for a minimum of 30 seconds. After one year of daily hanging, I have total flexibility with both shoulders, and I can do windmills, jumping jacks, yoga, archery, throw a football, swing a baseball bat, play tennis and golf, swim. you name it. And of course, I am working out with weights harder than ever, knowing that my shoulders have been remodeled. Talk about a miracle!"

* * * * *

2015 Peter   Makes so much sense!

As a CrossFit coach and weightlifting coach and a lifetime athlete I struggle with shoulder pain. I always thought this was normal and would be solved by itself. With this book I realize that that gravity plus bad positions can create SIS (subacromial impingement). Being a pragmatic, I am not so interested in the science but rather practical applications on how to solve my problem. This book provides exactly that. Hanging from a bar and lifting light weights overhead is the solution. Protocol could be 3 times a week (at least) hang 30 seconds 6 times and 30 repetitions of lateral, frontal raises with 4lb weights. Something like that. This makes total sense considering that our species used to live in trees and used hanging and swinging in them (brachiatinig) which solved this gravity/position automatically. Great easy read. Implement hanging in your life now!

* * * * *

2016 JH 2016 "Don't trust your doctor, buy this book and relieve your shoulder pain free and never have surgery."

xl

"If you have shoulder pain get this book. If you have scheduled shoulder surgery Get This Book Now! You will cancel your surgery. In my estimation you will never need surgery if you use this book. I was scheduled for left shoulder surgery and went through with it. The pain from it was still hurting after 2 years and now the other shoulder I'm told, my right, needs surgery. Then I found this book. I began the exercises and now not only do I not need another surgery on the right shoulder but the left that had been operated on and was hurting for over 2 years is pain free! A new shoulder is completely OUT OF THE QUESTION NOW! Do not hesitate as this will be one of the most valuable books you own. Why don't all doctors tell you this rather than do surgery? GET THIS BOOK NOW!"

* * * * *

2017 Araribat

"This was a long overdue review (bought this book back in 2013) and I'm taking the time now to write it because I owe it to the author and the public to share my experience and the results I got from following the instructions in this book. As mentioned already, based on the five-star rating, the instructions in this book helped me fix my right shoulder pain, which was caused by a tear in the rotator cuff. About 3 or 4 weeks into the daily sessions, I started noticing a definite improvement in the pain level. A few weeks into faithfully doing the workout the pain started subsiding noticeably. At that point I fully bought into it. As I only had a small tear in my rotator cuff and perhaps that worked in my favor with my injury not being very serious. Since not every shoulder injury is the same, it may or may not work for you, but I recommend you try it. Practically no cost other than the contraption you can buy in the fitness/sports sections of stores or build yourself using materials from your local hardware store. Hope this helps."

* * * * *

2009 Dale S.

"I was having a lot of pain in my right shoulder. I decided to go to an orthopedic surgeon. They did an MRI and the results were a torn rotator cuff. They said I needed surgery as soon as possible. It was my busy season so I was going to have to put it off until Sept. or Oct. I believe this was May 2006. Sometime during the next month or two I ran into Dr. Kirsch. I told him about my shoulder problem. He said he didn't think I needed surgery. He told me to put up a bar in my

basement and hang from it as long as I could. He said it would hurt and it did. He said after that I should get two 5lb weights and lift them from the side of my body up over my head. In a matter of days my shoulder was feeling better. It wasn't very long and the pain was gone and still is. I have told a lot of people about Dr. Kirsch's method. In my experience Dr. Kirsch's cure was a lot better than the alternative. Thanks Dr. Kirsch."

* * * * *

2019 Lee "Finally an exercise program that works for my injured shoulder."

"I've had shoulder pain for the past 20 years. About 5 years ago, I really aggravated my left shoulder while kayak surfing (an overextended paddle brace into a wave). Since then, I've seen numerous doctors, chiropractors, physical therapists, massage therapists and an acupuncturist. I was told that I had shoulder bursitis or a rotator cuff tear. I had a cortisone shot, but nothing seemed to help other than shoulder stretch exercises.

I spoke to other guys at the gym about my shoulder pain. Several guys mentioned passive hanging, but I dismissed it since it didn't make sense to me how hanging could help my shoulder pain.

Last month I saw a YouTube video by physical therapists discussing cuff tears and other shoulder issues. That video led me to other YouTube videos touting the benefits of passive hanging so I tried it. After one week, I was pleasantly surprised to find that I was able to freestyle swim with significantly less pain than before so I ordered Dr. Kirsch's book. I also found that I had less pain and better range of motion when my arms were extended over my head.

"Shoulder Pain? The Solution & Prevention" isn't a long book or overly technical or medical for the layperson. It includes some testimonials from people who have benefited from passive hanging.

In the beginning, passive hanging will be painful and difficult, the benefits may not be noticeable unless you're consistently doing it. Some people have difficulty doing a passive dead-hang. I have arthritis in both my hands so my grip strength is weak so I do partial assisted passive hangs. I wish I had read this book many years ago."

* * * * *

2014 D. J.

"OMG! Went to a masseuse who did some good work. Saw a chiropractor who made it worse. Went to a Physio and that did nothing. My doc recommended an appt with a surgeon. In the meanwhile, as I waited for the surgical appt I studied this book and did the exercises. In a nutshell hang from a bar as long as you can stand it every single day - starting with as much weight as you can bear until you can hang your full bodyweight. After a week my frozen shoulder was better. A year later I'm writing this review and my shoulder is cured. DO NOT go for surgery until you have tried this book!!!!!"

* * * * *

2013 Richie (In the UK) "Incredible! If you have shoulder pain, buy this book."

"I had suffered from shoulder pain in my left shoulder for coming up to a year. Gradually worsening so I could no longer do press-ups, pull-ups, sit for even a short length of time at a PC, or lift weights above my head. I was about to see my GP when I discovered this book. I'm no medical expert, but what was written about shoulders, their anatomy and their problems made sense. I gave the exercises a go. The problem wasn't cured immediately (the book doesn't claim they would be) but you feel the benefit immediately. Now after about 3 months the pain is almost gone. I can now do push-ups and pull-ups and I would say my shoulder feels almost back to normal. Yes, you do need a bar to do the exercises, ideally one where you can hang full length-I use a chin up bar which is not ideal. But do not let that put you off. This book is literally amazing. Now I just need Mr. Kirsch to find a cure for knee pain!"

* * * * *

2018 David G.

"I am absolutely astounded at the results I have gotten from the exercise regime in this book. I have suffered from impingement issues with both shoulders for 3 to 4 years; an MRI revealed supraspinatus tendonitis and type 2 SLAP tears of the superior labrum. I had tried physical therapy, osteopathy, chiropractic treatment, cortisone injections and a host of other alternative treatments. None helped for very long at all. The hanging, perhaps aided by the other exercises, but certainly the hanging has left me pain-free for the first time in

years. I felt a benefit after the first time and by the end of the third day all pain and movement restriction were gone. At the moment I am hanging doing 3 circuits of his exercises, with a 15 second hang and 20 repetitions of each of the weight exercises with 2.5lbs. I am now back to being able to exercise with no issues for the first time in 4 years. Just for the record I am 47 years old."

* * * *

2016 S.T. "Magic!

"I was having pain in my upper arm and shoulder. I could not even fasten my bra without pain. I went to the orthopedist and he said I needed surgery for the rotator cuff. I am an avid golfer and am very active. I knew I would have a hard time enduring the long recovery from shoulder surgery. I tried what Dr. Kirsch said and my shoulder pain went away! I make sure I go to the gym three times a week and hang. It does not take long, but it is magical. I am so thankful I found out this method. It's a shame that orthopedists are so ready to cut and fail to offer this as an option to avoid surgery and fix many shoulder problems!"

* * * * *

2012 J.T. "Best Thing I've Found"

"Both my shoulders have been painful for at least two years. I'm 44 and have impingement syndrome. I've now done four full hanging sessions 8 minutes of hanging and it's already obvious that this is doing more than anything I've tried so far. The aim here is to re-shape your shoulders, and to that end one needs to be prepared to make hanging a part of your routine. I'll update in a couple months or so.

Well, now it's over a year later and my enthusiasm for hanging as the basis for curing impingement syndrome is stronger than ever, my shoulders are almost healed. I can swim front crawl up to about five miles a week. I'm still hanging and don't plan to stop. I had six weeks away from home and that caused a lot of trouble. Decreased range of motion, more impingement pain, etc. Three days after resuming hanging most of the damage has been reversed and I'm back on track. This is something we should do for the rest of one's life-no gimmicks here-but it is an enormously powerful form of therapy. For goodness sake, don't gripe about the price of the book. If you have shoulder and arm trouble Dr. Kirsch's ideas are hard to put a value on. I'm deeply grateful to the man."

* * * * *

2019 R.K. Wow!

I had frozen shoulder condition about a year ago. I could barely put on a shirt or jacket. Could not wash my under arms in the shower. Could hardly reach to grab something from the fridge without pain. My trap muscle would trigger sharp pains all day long. My neck was so bad I could not turn my head to back out of the driveway. I could go on. I was using a heating pad several hours a day and many different portable massagers just to get through the day. I bought a pull up bar and started doing the hanging exercise six months ago. At first I had to use my right arm to lift my left arm onto the bar, it hurt like hell to do it, but the book explains that. For the first week I could only stand 30 seconds at a time, for 5 or 6 times a day. I could tell it was helping because I was beginning to be able to sleep for longer periods of time. I next bought an LED timer so I could see exactly how long I was hanging and it encouraged me to try to hang longer each day. I finally got to 2 and then 3 and now 5 minutes each session. Now I do two 5 minutes sessions every morning and 1 or 2 during the day if needed. My shoulders have not felt this good in years. I have almost no neck pain anymore. I can sleep on my side all night with no pain. This is something I'll be doing for the rest of my life. When I think about how bad I was and how if I had gone to the doctor and what they would have done to me I cannot be more grateful to the good doctor for publishing this book. I have bought 4 copies for my friends.

* * * * *

Those who have made the effort to use the hanging exercise have usually been rewarded with prompt and lasting relief. For those interested in reading more testimonials, many more reviews are available at Amazon books. For even more evidence as to the success of the program simply go to the internet and search for "hanging for shoulder pain." You will find numerous references to the book you are reading. Or go to www.kirschshoulder.com, or search YouTube with Dr. John M. Kirsch.

PART ONE
The Enigma of the Shoulder

My Story:
Solving the Enigma of the Shoulder

In the late 1970s I was performing many knee arthroscopies in my orthopedic practice. In those years we did not have the luxury of miniature video cameras. Instead we were required to sit at the foot of the table looking through an arthroscope while holding the scope up with the arms elevated for long hours. By the early 1980s I had developed severe impingement (subacromial impingement or SIS) pain in both shoulders from the long hours in the operating room, and I puzzled over what to do. Then I stumbled upon an idea that changed my life.

I was hiking in a park with my two young boys when we came upon a horizontal ladder. The boys climbed to the ladder and swung across like little monkeys. Then it was my turn. As I reached for the second rung of the ladder the shoulder pain was immediate and I realized I would never reach it. And then I sensed that the reason I could not do the ladder was because I had not been doing it! I had not been hanging or brachiating. If you want to be able to do something you must do it. If you want to run a marathon, you must run and run and run. The same is true of the shoulder. If you want to be able to use your arm for overhead activity you must use the arm for overhead activity. In the words of F.J. Kottke [1], a noted exercise physiologist:

"**Normal motion** in joints and soft tissue is maintained by **normal movement** of the parts of the body which elongate and stretch joint capsules, muscles, subcutaneous tissues, and ligaments through the full range of motion many times each day." It was just intuition. *I decided that if I were to hang from a bar it would compress the swollen subacromial bursa tissues and re-shape the CA arch that compresses the rotator cuff.*

3

Without overhead arm activity the space between the acromion and the humerus undergoes slow contracture resulting in degenerative changes.

The evidence teaches us that as humans we must simulate brachiating by frequent hanging from a bar and doing light weight lifting. I also sensed that the hanging exercise might be the solution to mid-life shoulder pain. Being an orthopedic surgeon with knowledge of the anatomy helped with this insight. I reasoned that if I could reshape and strengthen my shoulder anatomy by hanging I might be able to avoid surgery.

I installed a bar from some ceiling beams and began hanging as long as I could. Initially I could only hang for a few seconds, but as time went on, I was able to hang for longer and longer periods. Even after a few days my shoulders began feeling better. At the beginning of each daily session the first effort to hang was painful. But 15-30 seconds into the exercise I noticed that the pain had stopped. When I returned to the bar each repetition became easier and easier.

Then I began lifting 5lb dumbbells to strengthen the rotator cuff tendons and muscles. At first this was painful and I could only lift a 5lb dumbbell about 20 times. After a week or two I had much less pain and after about 3 months my shoulder pain was gone and I could lift an 8lb dumbbell doing 50 repetitions in each of three directions.

Then thirty years ago I was bowled over by two large dogs and I suffered a complete tear of my rotator cuff. An MRI showed that the supraspinatus tendon was completely torn and the muscle retracted. So now I had both the subacromial impingement syndrome and a torn rotator cuff. I could not lift my arm. But after several weeks I once again began the painful process of hanging from the overhead bar and trying to lift light weights.

This exercise was accompanied by painful crunching and grinding in the shoulder. Initially I could barely lift the arm to the horizon. Then I attached some elastic bands to the ceiling and used them to pull my arm up. I gradually began helping the elastic bands lift my arm. This gradually strengthened my arm and after some months of hanging and weight lifting I could lift a 10lb weight 150 times to a full overhead position each day. I was once again able to play tennis with a strong accurate serve using the arm with the large rotator cuff tear.

I believe this story of my recovery is best explained by the redundancy built into the human body. Other muscles can substitute for the lost function of the injured parts. Nature provides us with backups.

Having had this personal success with the exercises I began incorporating them into my practice and recommending them for patients. These exercises have helped many people avoid therapy and shoulder surgery.

The cost of medical care in the United States is astounding. In 2018 the annual estimated cost of musculoskeletal care in the U.S. was more than $300 billion. Musculoskeletal problems are one of the leading causes of disability in this country. Of these conditions, shoulder pain is the third most common disorder. There are 4.5 million doctor visits each year for shoulder pain.

The exercises that I used to heal my shoulders relieve most shoulder pain quickly, sometimes in days or several weeks. These exercises involve simply hanging from an overhead support such as an exercise bar and lifting dumbbell weights. All a person needs are a *"branch to hang from and a brick to lift."* It is that simple.

This book is not intended to be an academic discourse. Even as it is primarily written for the public, it is my hope that those healthcare workers treating persons with shoulder pain read and understand the information in this book. There are a few references to the scientific literature but I have kept these to a minimum. There is no other book that puts forth a hanging exercise to overcome the degenerative changes of the shoulder caused by age, gravity and disuse; or explains another joint in the shoulder, the acromiohumeral joint.

You will also find that much of the text and many of the images are repeated in different sections. This is deliberate and done for emphasis. The anatomy of the shoulder is complex and the medical terminology difficult for the average person so I have simplified the wording wherever possible.

The usual professional recommendations for relieving shoulder pain are rest, ice, anti-inflammatory drugs, various exercises considered safe because they do not increase the pain. When you seek care with your doctor for shoulder pain, he/she will usually make a diagnosis, order medication and refer you to a physical therapist. The physical therapist will initiate and supervise various treatments or what are called "modalities" such as the use of heat, vibration, or electric current applied to the shoulder area. They may apply cortisone to the skin, do massage or stretch your shoulder. Some safe stretching exercises will be ordered, but usually you will be advised to avoid pain while doing these exercise routines. Strengthening exercises will be ordered, but limited to weight lifting without raising your arm above the level that causes pain. After 2-3 weeks, you might be referred back to your doctor who will then order scans of your shoulder (usually expensive MRI studies) and may then recommend more physical therapy, pills, cortisone shots or surgery.

Part of the patient's problem is that they are overwhelmed with the sophistication of an MRI or CT scan. When the surgeon points out what he thinks is the problem on the scan, the patient is dazzled. Surgeons too often operate based on the findings on the x-ray, MRI or CT scan and their exam. They give the patient every opportunity to avoid surgery using therapy and medications, but these failing, they do their best to help the patient with surgery. Most patients become committed to surgery because they have "seen the tear" in real life imaging. What have you got to lose? Surgery versus the simple exercises in the book. The exercises are free.

What I just described is the usual available treatment for the shoulder. While some of these treatments are helpful, they usually require repeated visits to the therapist or physician and all too often do not solve the shoulder problem. Going through this medical routine is expensive and for many with shoulder pain unnecessary.

Why a hanging exercise has not been recommended in standard shoulder treatment programs is understandable. There has been no previous research conducted on a hanging exercise other than the study upon which this book is based. Surgeons will perform an expensive operation that removes a few mm of bone from the acromion and part of the bursa to make more room for the rotator cuff. This surgery removes important tissues from the acromiohumeral joint. The results of this expensive surgery are confusing at best. The hanging exercise will provide the same increase in "roominess" by remodeling or reshaping the shoulder bones and ligaments and by restoring the normal compliance/flexibility of these structures. Using the exercises you can usually avoid pills, therapy and surgery.

Judging from comments on the hanging exercise by some therapists and physicians it seems to be a common thought that you might injure the shoulder when you perform the hanging exercise. It is clear from more than 36 years of clinical research on the hanging exercise that it is not only safe, but extremely effective in relieving and preventing the most common causes of shoulder pain. Until I discovered the hanging exercise, I followed the usual physical-therapy-followed-by-surgery routine in my practice. Up until then, I had no alternative treatment options. After 1983 I became far more conservative and performed far fewer surgeries for the shoulder. Many of those who began the hanging exercise and weight lifting had relief from their pain within days or weeks of beginning the exercises.

A colleague added these thoughts:

"In his quest to relieve shoulder pain sufferers everywhere, Dr. Kirsch presents a method he found relieved and restored the motion in his shoulder after he fell and sustained a massive tear of his rotator cuff. When he asked for my opinion I strongly recommended immediate open repair of his rotator cuff. One year later I saw Dr. Kirsch and asked how his shoulder was doing. He demonstrated full range of motion. I was astounded and asked who had done the surgery. He answered, 'No one. I just did my hanging and weight lifting exercises.' I thought it was a fluke. But then he showed me others who had followed his hanging protocol and read testimonials at Amazon. More and more it has become my preferential way to manage shoulders. The number of people Dr. Kirsch helped avoid surgery is staggering. To date, therapists and surgeons have dismissed the exercises in the book. Give it a try, what have you got to lose? It's Free!"

As the Twig is Bent:
How the Shoulder is Remodeled by Hanging

A tree may be reshaped by bending and training its branches. The secret to the most common shoulder problem, the subacromial impingement syndrome (SIS), is that the contracted CA arch tissues can be stretched and reshaped by hanging. This we know from a number of facts:

Bone and other tissues will be reshaped as a result of stresses applied to the tissue. It is the same principle that Orthodontists rely on to straighten teeth. This principle is called **Wolff's Law** [2].

We know from laboratory cadaver experiments that the acromion will bend and the coracoacromial ligament will stretch when the arm is lifted by a force

In these experiments strain gauges were placed in the acromion bone of the CA arch to measure the bending [3]. **It is this acromial bending that maintains the health of the shoulder.** Repeated prolonged bending and stretching employing Wolff's Law will reshape these structures, providing more room for the rotator cuff.

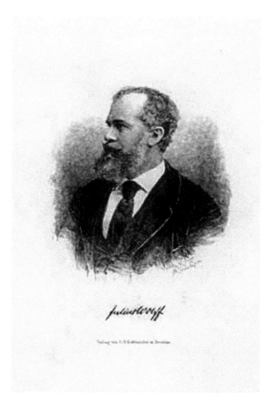

Fig. 19 Julius Wolff (1836–1902). Wolff's Law is a theory developed by Wolff, a German anatomist and surgeon, in the 19th century; which states that "bone in a healthy person or animal will adapt to the loads under which it is placed."

Beginnings of Shoulder Problems

The gradual shrinking of the subacromial space due to time and neglect leads to friction, wear and tear and eventually tears of the rotator cuff. Hanging will bend the acromion and stretch the coracoacromial ligament increasing the space in which the rotator cuff tendons can move without obstruction. This is the mechanism by which the shoulder is healed.

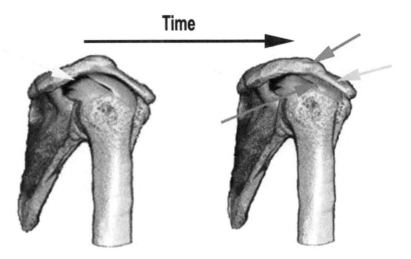

Fig. 20 This is how the CA arch becomes deformed by neglecting to hang or brachiate. Over time, with gravity and disuse, the acromion becomes deformed in a downward direction into a hooked shape and the coracoacromial ligament shortens. These deformities press on the rotator cuff tendons causing inflammation and pain. Pink arrow, inflamed rotator cuff tendons; red arrow, hooked deformity of the acromion; green arrow, shortened coracoacromial ligament; yellow arrow, the subacromial space.

A Little Shoulder Anatomy

I do not go into great detail describing shoulder anatomy as in shoulder textbooks. The hanging exercise makes understanding every aspect of the anatomy unnecessary. The exercise heals and maintains the shoulder in most cases regardless of the diagnosis.

X-rays

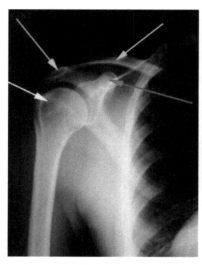 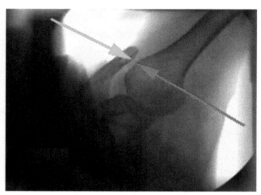

Fig. 21   **Fig. 22**

Fig. 21 X-ray. Yellow arrow, humerus; green arrow, acromion; red arrow, coracoid process; orange arrow, the clavicle.

Fig. 22 Image taken from an x-ray video of a subject raising the arm to show the acromiohumeral joint. The space between the arrows constitutes the acromiohumeral joint. This will be explained repeatedly throughout the book. Green arrow, acromion; red arrow, the humerus.

The New Joint in the Shoulder
The Acromiohumeral Joint

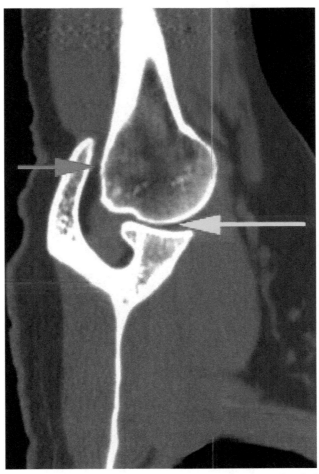

Fig. 23 A sagittal slice view of the two main joints in the shoulder: red arrow the new joint in the shoulder, the acromiohumeral joint, green arrow: the glenohumeral joint.

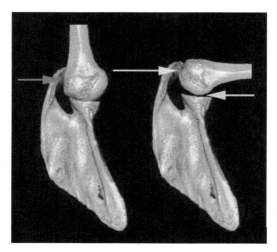

Fig. 24 On the left, 3D image of the shoulder while hanging, red arrow, the acromiohumeral joint. On the right, when the arm is lowered the acromio-humeral joint is no longer engaged. Gold arrow, space for rotator cuff tendons; green arrow, the glenohumeral joint.

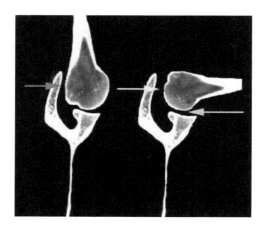

Fig. 25 The same anatomy as in **Fig. 24** in a sagittal slice image. Red arrow, the acromiohumeral joint. On the left, the humerus leans on and bends the acromion.

The Usual Presentation of Shoulder Anatomy

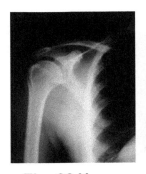 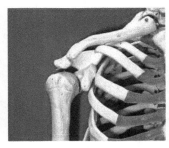 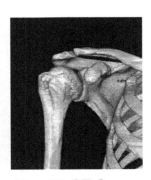

Fig. 26 X-ray. **Fig. 27** Skeleton. **Fig. 28** CT Scan.

This common presentation of the shoulder, arm at the side, prevents us from having a more complete understanding of shoulder biomechanics.

The Skeleton Seen While Hanging

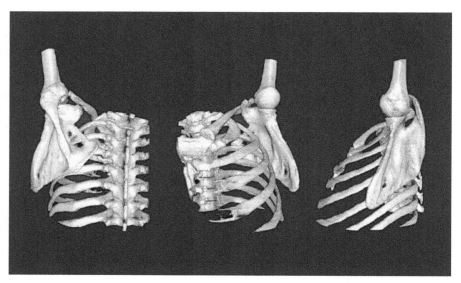

Fig. 29 Shoulder skeleton shown during simulation of the hanging exercise. Viewing these images of the shoulder skeleton made while simulating the hanging exercise gives us a new insight into the biomechanics of the shoulder. There is no other source that presents these views of the shoulder. Search the web for an image of the shoulder skeleton seen while hanging. There are none.

The Scapulothoracic Joint

An important aspect of the shoulder is the scapulothoracic (ST) joint. The space between the scapula and the ribs is the scapulothoracic joint. This joint is formed by the scapula (shoulder blade) gliding around on the thorax or chest. The wide range of motion available to the shoulder is due in large part to the range of movement available at this joint. You can view scapulothoracic joint motion videos on YouTube.

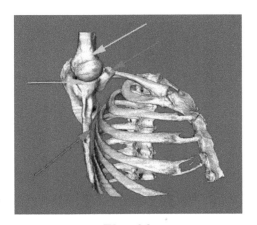
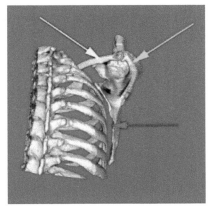

Fig. 30   **Fig. 31**

An important aspect of the shoulder: the scapulothoracic (ST) joint — red arrows. The space between the scapula and the ribs is the ST joint. This joint is formed by the scapula (shoulder blade) gliding around on the thorax (chest) with interposed muscles providing the lubrication.

In **Fig. 30**, Front/anterior view: red arrow, the scapulothoracic joint; green arrow, the humerus; gold arrow, the glenohumeral joint; pink arrow, the coracoid process. In **Fig. 31**, Back/posterior view: red arrow, scapulothoracic joint; yellow arrow, clavicle; green arrow, acromion. The scapulothoracic joint is also termed an articulation or scapulothoracic interface.

Shoulder Muscles and Tendons

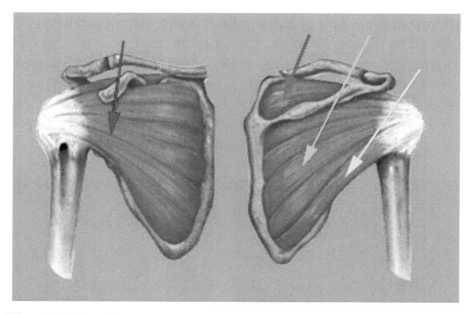

Fig. 32 The four rotator cuff muscles and tendons. On left, anterior/front view: blue arrow, **subscapularis**. On right, posterior/rear view: red arrow, **supraspinatus**; green arrow, **infraspinatus**; yellow arrow, **teres minor**. These muscles elevate the arm and keep the ball of the humerus in the glenoid socket. Image adapted from the web.

Acromial Shapes

There is a classification of different shapes of the acromion in the literature that is arbitrary. Acromial shapes lie on a continuum from less hooking to more hooking, but all will bend and remodel when one hangs.

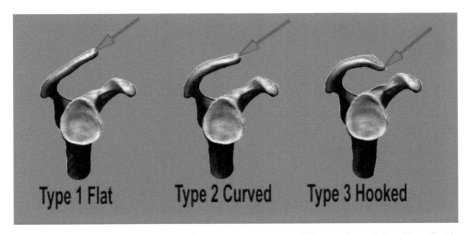

Fig. 33 Red arrows, the acromion. The "hooking" of the acromion shown is probably exaggerated. Image adapted from the web.

The acromial shape varies from flat Type 1, to curved Type 2, to hooked Type 3. No matter what the degree of hooking, the hanging exercise will, in time, bend the acromion decreasing the hooking and relieve the subacromial impingement (SIS) preventing rotator cuff tears. Research has shown that the different shapes of the acromion are acquired as a response to traction forces applied via the coracoacromial ligament (CAL) and are not present at birth. Surgeons commonly operate to remove the hooked part of the acromion doing what's called a "subacromial decompression surgery (SAD)."

Cadaver Shoulder View

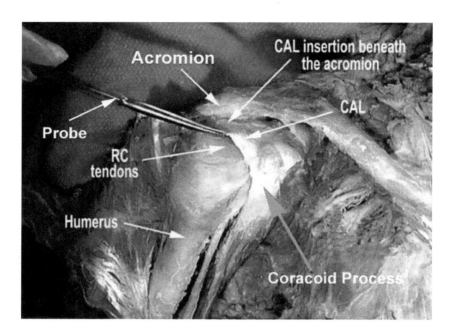

Fig. 34 A cadaver view showing the CA arch: acromion, CAL (coracoacromial ligament) and the coracoid process, orange arrow (see the "CA Arch" **Fig. 3 & 68**). A probe has been placed beneath the coracoacromial ligament to lift this structure for demonstration. Notice that the ligament inserts on the *undersurface* of the acromion. This position of the CAL allows it to provide a gliding surface for the rotator cuff tendons that lie beneath the ligament. During subacromial decompression surgery (SAD), the CAL ligament is excised or released removing this important structure that cushions and lubricates the acromiohumeral joint. If the CAL is deformed by time, gravity and disuse, the ligament may cause subacromial impingement and rotator cuff damage.

CT Scan Images While Hanging

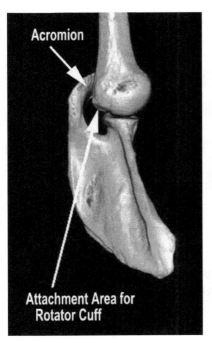

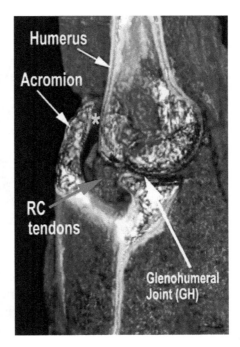

Fig. 35   **Fig. 36**

The images taken from a CT scan of a subject simulating the hanging position. In **Fig. 35** one can see the relationship of the humerus and scapula while hanging. In **Fig. 36** the rotator cuff (RC) tendons and muscles are relaxed in their "position of rest." This image was made with a CT setting to show soft tissue. Note the position of the rotator cuff tendons. The tendons and their insertions on the humerus (red arrow) are well away from the acromion. This position of the rotator cuff tendons makes it impossible to injure these tendons during the hanging exercise. The green asterisk marks the acromiohumeral joint. The humerus leaning on the acromion gradually bends the acromion creating more room for the rotator cuff tendons. These images are seen in videos at www.kirschshoulder.com and YouTube at Dr. John M. Kirsch.

Acromiohumeral Joint Close-up View

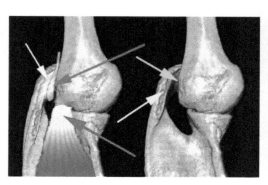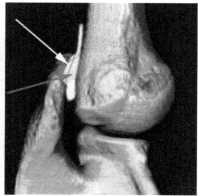

| **Fig. 37** | **Fig. 38** |

These images demonstrate the joint between the humerus and the acromion, the "acromiohumeral joint" (green arrow) and the artist's rendering of the soft tissues between these two bony parts of the shoulder. These soft tissues include the coracoacromial ligament (CAL) (white arrows) as it inserts on the undersurface of the acromion, the subacromial bursa (pink arrows), and the rotator cuff tendons and muscles (red arrow). Note the safe positioning of the rotator cuff tendon insertions (red arrow). The tendons and their insertions are well behind the acromion that could pinch or injure the tendons. Acromion (yellow arrow).

The Exercises

Who Should Do the Exercises?

Everyone should do these exercises; because not only do the exercises relieve most shoulder pain problems, they prevent them from occurring.

We humans, along with some of the apes, (gibbon, siamang, and occasionally the orangutan, gorilla and chimpanzee) possess the unique innate ability to hang by our hands, or to "brachiate." Like it or not, we humans, if healthy, and some of the apes share very similar shoulder anatomy and prehensile function, i.e.; the ability to grasp a bar or tree limb and swing from bar to bar, limb to limb.

As children we hung from monkey bars and similar playground equipment. Infants are capable of hanging from various supports. Moving on from childhood most of us turn to other activities including various sports. Very few sport activities require brachiating or hanging. Thus, in time we lose this facility that we were given at birth. Even so, most otherwise healthy persons if motivated, are capable of regaining the ability to simulate brachiating by hanging from a bar. If they could only find one. Look around, it will be difficult to find something from which to hang. Suitable hanging bars have been removed from most playgrounds and are not provided in most gyms.

The exercises described here are for those who want to relieve their subacromial impingement syndrome (SIS), rotator cuff injury or frozen shoulder and maintain healthy shoulders without pills, therapy or surgery. The exercises may be used even in the presence of rotator cuff tears. If you can lift the arm to the horizon with good strength, you should be able to begin the exercises. If the arm can be lifted to the horizon, the rotator cuff will not be further pinched or irritated by the exercises. These exercises are for persons of all walks and ages of life; whether you are a business man, laborer, athlete, man or woman.

The athlete who uses the shoulder for overhead activity will find the hanging exercise very helpful in relieving and preventing further shoulder problems. Swimmers, football, hockey, baseball, tennis and basketball players all depend on painless repeated arm elevation for their sport. The exercises described in this book will insure maximal freedom and strength with repeated arm elevation.

The causes of shoulder pain have been extensively studied but remain poorly understood. It has been established that certain work conditions are more likely to result in shoulder pain. Prolonged overhead work, heavy loads, pushing, pulling, and sustained arm elevation such as in hairdressers.

The typical person that will use the hanging exercise is otherwise healthy but has shoulder pain that appears for no apparent reason. They might suddenly notice that putting on a coat causes pain in the shoulder, or sitting at their computer they begin having pain in the shoulder holding the mouse, or doing overhead work of any sort causes shoulder pain. Others may find that their shoulders begin to feel stiff and have pain that limits their range of motion. Intermittent stretching and hanging from a support will relieve the pain associated with prolonged computer/desk work.

The hanging exercise will not relieve all shoulder ailments. The exercise will stretch the arch of ligament and bone covering the rotator cuff, the CA arch that consists of the acromion, the coracoacromial ligament (CAL) and the coracoid process, and compress the swollen subacromial bursa thus maintaining the health of these tissues. There are many other parts of the body that are stretched during a hanging exercise including the spine.

The Hanging Exercise

The first and by far the most important exercise that will relieve shoulder pain by reshaping the bone and ligaments that pinch the rotator cuff is hanging from an overhead bar. This is the *only* shoulder exercise that will effectively stretch, bend and reshape the CA arch to provide more room for the rotator cuff. If you already know that you have a tear of your rotator cuff from an MRI study or some other tests, the hanging exercise will not worsen the tear. While hanging, the rotator cuff is relaxed and far behind the offending CA arch.

Be sure to remove any hand jewelry that might interfere with hanging onto the bar (rings, etc.). Weight lifting hooks that strap to the wrist may allow longer hanging times. As you progress with your hanging program, you will notice that calluses will form on your fingers and palms. This is a normal response to the hanging exercise but may be diminished using gloves and bar padding.

The hanging exercise is done over a 10- to 15-minute period during which you hang for 10- to 30-second intervals using both hands as tolerated, applying full or partial body weight. You should hang for brief intervals at first, taking rest breaks for a minute or so. While hanging, the shoulders and body should be relaxed allowing gravity to act on the shoulder muscles, bones and ligaments. Allow gravity to do its job. The only body parts which should be active are the hands for gripping the bar. The hands must be in a position with the palms facing forward, not in the chin-up position. The chin-up arm position will not stretch the CA arch as in this position the arm cannot be raised high enough to apply a bending force to the CA arch. Full arm elevation occurs only while hanging with the palms forward. To test this try raising your arm palm up and then palm down.

Most persons will have a fair amount of pain or discomfort when first attempting to hang. The exercise is in this sense counter-intuitive, or paradoxical. Paradoxically, the pain experienced while hanging from a bar will not injure the shoulder, but must be accepted to overcome the contracture of the CA arch and stiffness of the scapular restraints. You will notice that the pain will subside after hanging for a few moments. If you do not have pain while hanging, the exercise is still important to reverse and prevent contracture of the CA arch.

Remind yourself that when you are hanging you are:

S-T-R-E-T-C-H-I-N-G

the CA arch. You have taken the first step in reshaping the shoulder. On the next pages are pictures of people doing the hanging exercise using bars and even a tree limb, nature's hanging bar!

People Hanging

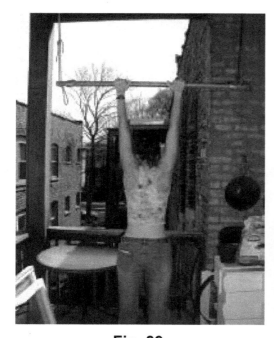

Fig. 39

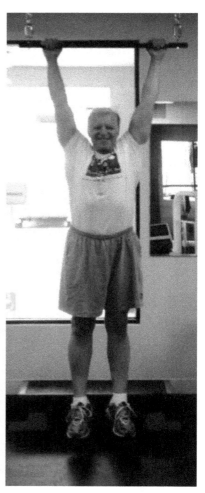

Fig. 40

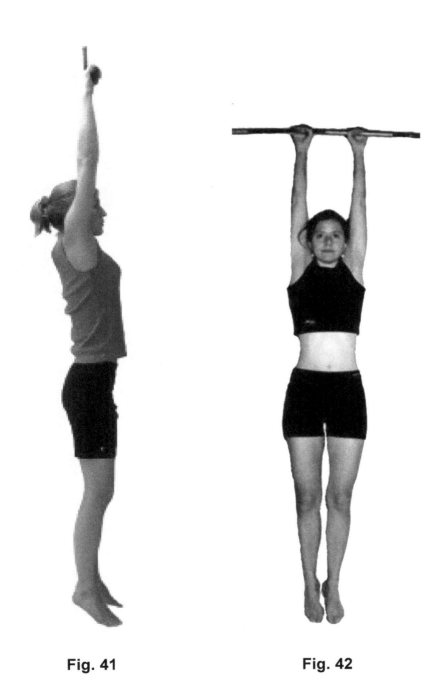

Fig. 41   Fig. 42

29

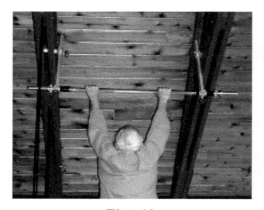
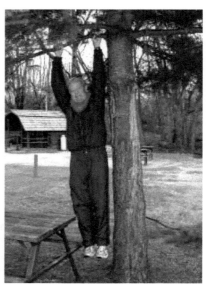

Fig. 43   **Fig. 44**

In **Fig. 43** the author hangs from a bar; and in **Fig. 44** from a handy tree.

Partial/Reduced Weight Hanging

At first you may not be able to hang with full body weight. You may begin by keeping your feet on the floor and grasping the bar positioned lower, and stretch by "partial" hanging until strength and reach improve.

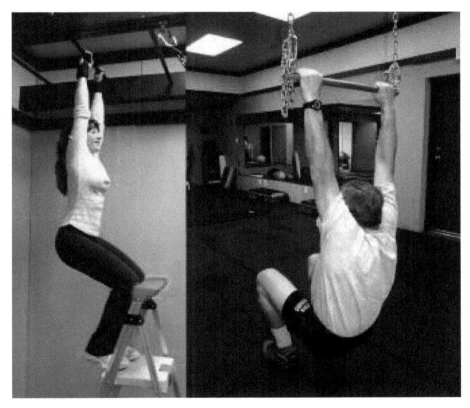

Fig. 45 Left: A fitness instructor demonstrates partial hanging using a support ladder. Right: A client hangs while squatting.

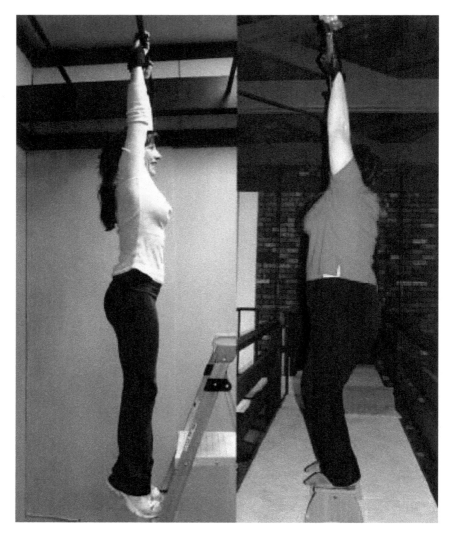

Fig. 46 Left: A physical fitness director demonstrates full hanging using a ladder to reach the overhead bar. Right: This subject healed **35** years of shoulder pain in two weeks with the partial weight hanging exercise.

Lifting Weights

The hanging exercise is followed with weight lifting exercises that are best performed immediately after the hanging exercise; for it is then that the CA arch has been stretched allowing the rotator cuff tendons to move more freely beneath the arch. These simple weight lifting exercises are important for strengthening the rotator cuff muscles and other muscles that raise the arm. Strengthening these muscles will balance the forces around the shoulder and restore the rotator cuff tendons and muscles to a robust healthy condition. The weight lifting exercises require more discipline than the hanging exercise. Hanging from an overhead bar is largely a passive exercise employing only the fingers to grasp the bar. Lifting weights, on the other hand, requires the active synchronous use of many muscles about the shoulder- the rotator cuff muscles, the latissimus dorsi, triceps, biceps, deltoid and other muscles. This requires work and discipline!

The weight lifting program is begun when one is able to raise the arm above the horizon with no added weight. Dumbbell weights of 1 to 8 pounds are used, doing as many repetitions and weight as tolerated. A realistic long-term goal for most persons is 30 to 45 repetitions. These exercises should include forward, lateral and extension arm elevations with the arm positioned with the palms down and brought to full elevation with each repetition. The palms down position is important, as it positions the upper part of the humerus bone to contact and stretch the CA arch ligament and bone.

If you already know that you have a rotator cuff tear but can lift the arm to the horizon, you may begin the hanging exercise and as time goes on, add the weight lifting exercises. By lifting lighter weights, doing fewer repetitions and avoiding arcs of motion that are painful, you should be able to work around the area of the rotator cuff tear and strengthen the parts of the rotator cuff that are still intact and healthy. Small rotator cuff tears may heal once the CA arch is stretched and remodeled by hanging. The weight lifting exercises are shown on the next pages.

Model Lifting Weights

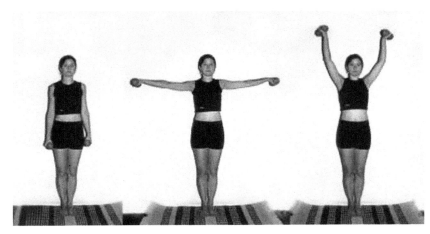

Fig. 47 The side weight lifting exercise. Your goal is to do 30–45 repetitions at any weight before increasing the weight of the dumbbell. Note the palms down position.

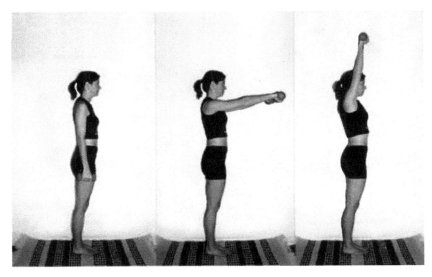

Fig. 48 The forward weight lifting exercise. Your goal is to do 30–45 repetitions at any weight before increasing the weight of the dumbbell. Note the palms down position.

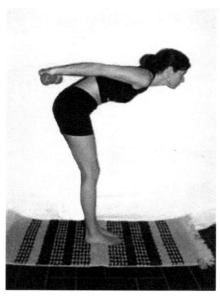

Fig. 49 The extension weight lifting exercise. In this exercise, the weights are brought from an arm at the side position backward and upward into extension as high as possible. Your goal is to do 30–45 repetitions at any weight before increasing the weight of the dumbbell. Note the palms must face the floor.

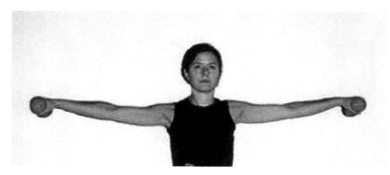

Fig. 50 Note the palms-down position of the hands while lifting weights. This position allows the side of the humerus to lift and stretch the CA arch. Take your time with the program, and after some months go by vary the program so that it will not become a boring routine. A video showing a model demonstrating the weight lifting exercise may be viewed on YouTube under John M. Kirsch and on our website www.kirschshoulder.com.

The palms forward position while hanging, and the palms down while lifting weights is of utmost importance. Try this on yourself: attempt lifting your arm with the palm up; then with the palm down. You will immediately notice that you are able to lift your arm to maximum height having your palm down. This puts your arm in the optimal position to lift and bend your acromion thus remodeling your own shoulder. Doing these two exercises, hanging from a bar and weight lifting should require only 15–20 minutes of your time each day. When the shoulder symptoms decrease, the exercises may be performed less often (perhaps only 2–3 times each week), but intermittent hanging and weight lifting should be continued as a life habit. Do not be in a hurry to progress with the exercises. Take your time, but keep at it. Remodeling the tissues will continue for many years after you begin the program. Over time, you will find that your weight lifting need not be so regimented, and you will develop your own pattern. As an example, perhaps you might lift in only one direction one day, and the next day another direction. Perhaps your weight lifting will be performed only a few times each week. Listen to your body and follow its advice. Patience and Persistence!

The Most Common Shoulder Problems

The rotator cuff is a complex of tendons in the shoulder that help lift the arm. Most rotator cuff tears are caused by the subacromial impingement syndrome (SIS), age and neglect. The impingement syndrome or subacromial pain syndrome is caused by tightness or contracture of the arch of ligament and bone (the CA arch) that covers the upper arm and rotator cuff tendons that lift the arm. This tightness or contracture of the CA arch is said to cause painful and destructive pinching of the rotator cuff. The cause of the contracture of the CA arch is uncertain, but most likely related to age, disuse (neglecting to hang, brachiate) and gravity. The average human arm weighs about 10lb. The continual pull of gravity on the arm, transferred through ligaments and muscles, may very gradually cause the CA arch to become deformed in a downward direction ultimately pinching the rotator cuff that is already weakened by disuse.

The Subacromial Impingement Syndrome (SIS) in the USA

The SubAcromial Pain Syndrome (SAPS) in Europe

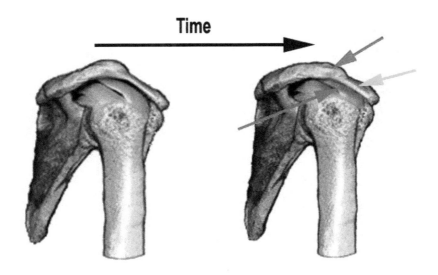

Fig. 51 The "subacromial impingement syndrome," more appropriately named "subacromial pain syndrome." On the left, image of a normal shoulder showing the rotator cuff tendons beneath the normal acromion and CA arch. On the right, due to time and neglect, the acromion becomes hooked (red arrow) pressing on the rotator cuff tendons that become inflamed (pink arrow) and the coracoacromial ligament (green arrow) is shortened.

Relieving the Impingement by Hanging

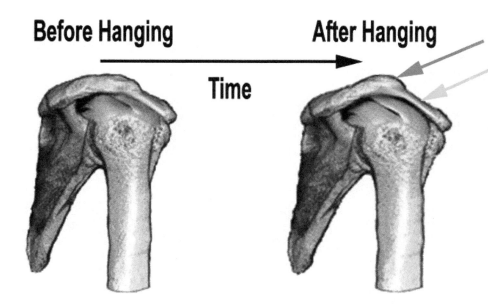

Before Hanging   **After Hanging**

Time

Fig. 52 There are no empty spaces in the shoulder tissues. Because of this compact structure of the shoulder tissues, the deformity of the acromion needn't be very large to cause problems: pain and irritating compression of the rotator cuff and tears. Perhaps it is because of this compact design of these structures that the hanging exercise, using the humerus leaning on the acromion, is able to efficiently bend the acromion back to a normal configuration relieving the subacromial impingement.

Acromial bending by hanging needn't be very large to relieve the shoulder pain. Compressing the subacromial bursa and bending the acromion only a few millimeters will relieve the subacromial impingent process and begin healing the shoulder without surgery. This is why many have relieved their shoulder pain within days of beginning the exercises.

The most popular shoulder surgery is arthroscopic or open subacromial decompression (SAD) with removal of part of the acromion and excision/release of the coracoacromial ligament. What happens during this surgery? First the acromion is shaved down to make more room for the rotator cuff tendons. Traditionally surgeons removed or released the coracoacromial ligament believing it gave better results. Now it is believed the ligament should be saved to prevent shoulder joint instability and now this is a topic of debate. The subacromial bursa is partially or completely removed.

I present the following studies to help you make an informed decision about having this surgery. Recent studies have called into question whether the surgery is really necessary or effective. The first arthroscopic subacromial decompression was performed in 1983. Its popularity has grown exponentially since then. Most available study reviews are from Europe and the UK.

A study in Great Britain (UK) recorded 2,523 surgeries in 2000, and 21,355 in 2010 and ten times that many in the United States. **A careful study of a large sample of the surgeries showed that there was no significant benefit from the operation.**

In another report, I cite a study presented in Barcelona, Spain in 2016. The group studied 140 patients who had arthroscopic subacromial decompression. After 12 years the results compared to those having no surgery showed that there was **no benefit from the operation. The group could not recommend surgery for subacromial impingement.** They recommended a structured exercise program rather than surgery.

In the BMJ (British Medical Journal) in February 2019 an article was published showing that the subacromial decompression surgery was found to be accompanied by serious complications including frozen shoulder, death, major bleeding, acromial fracture, deep infection, peripheral nerve injuries, venous thromboembolism and serious anesthesia complications; and that **there was essentially no benefit from the surgery.** While real, the incidence of these complications is low, less than 3%. **The study panel concluded that almost all well-informed patients would decline surgery and therefore made a strong recommendation against the surgery.**

In the United States, a study done in February 2019 and published in the Journal of Bone and Joint Surgery, it was found that there was no difference between simple diagnostic shoulder arthroscopy and arthroscopic subacromial decompression surgery. The findings did not support the current practice of performing subacromial decompression on all patients with shoulder impingement syndrome.

There have been many other outcome studies performed to evaluate the success of subacromial decompression surgery and the results are confusing at best. Considering the ordeal of having surgery and the protracted months of therapy, its startling cost ($25,000.00+ average in 2019) with its dubious success rate, the hanging exercise with a near 90% success would seem preferable. After the surgery, it cannot be undone, and no one can give you back your shoulder.

Authorities claim that the impingement syndrome is caused by overuse or wear and tear and that repeated use of the shoulder can make the tendons swell, causing them to "catch" on the acromion. They also suggest that the sport activities that most likely lead to "impingement" are swimming, tennis, basketball, football, baseball, wrestling and hockey. Occupations that increase your risk are construction work, moving heavy boxes and painting. My studies suggest that it is not overuse that is to blame for the impingement, but rather disuse. By neglecting to hang, or brachiate, the acromion becomes deformed and pinches the rotator cuff and subacromial bursa causing inflammation and pain.

The Subacromial Decompression Surgery (SAD)

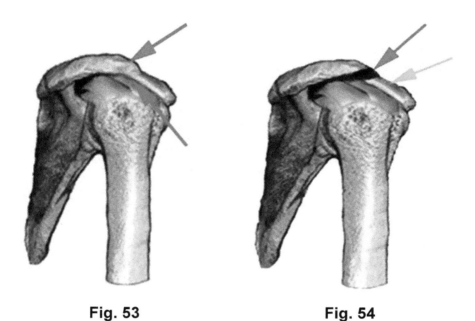

Fig. 53   **Fig. 54**

Fig. 53 Over time, the acromion (red arrow) has become hooked pressing on the rotator cuff tendons below causing inflammation and pain (pink arrow).

Fig. 54 When subacromial decompression (SAD) surgery is performed, the hooked part of the acromion (red arrow) and part of the coracoacromial ligament are removed (green arrow). This causes damage to these important components of the shoulder and produces instability of the coracoacromial arch. When the hooked part of the acromion is removed and the coracoacromial ligament detached or excised, the acromion is weakened and may fracture during post-surgical physical therapy. Disability is often permanent.

The Kirsch Institute Theory:
The Hanging Exercise Relieves the Subacromial Impingement Syndrome/Subacromial Pain Syndrome Without Surgery

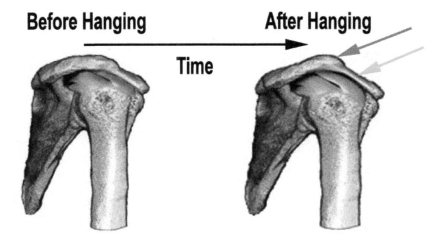

Fig. 55 The hanging exercise over time corrects the hooked acromion and stretches the coracoacromial ligament (CAL) without damaging the acromion or the coracoacromial ligament thus healing the subacromial impingement without pills, therapy or surgery. Red arrow, the acromion is restored making more room for the rotator cuff tendons relieving the inflammation; green arrow, the coracoacromial ligament is lengthened to normal.

The Torn Rotator Cuff

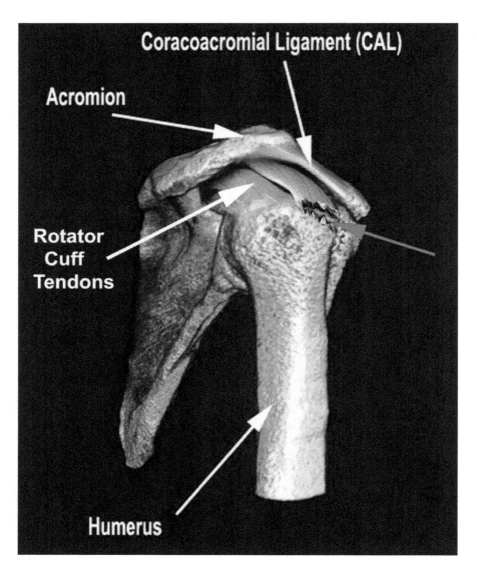

Fig. 56 After years of neglect, the impingement process may eventually cause tears in the rotator cuff. Red arrow, a rotator cuff tear. Artist's rendering.

The causes of a rotator cuff tear are said to be almost the same as the causes of the impingement syndrome. Excessive repetitive overhead use of the arm as in swimming, baseball, hockey, basketball, tennis, football, and wrestling and any occupation that requires the same repetitive overhead arm use. My studies suggest the opposite. Avoidance of overhead use of the arm or hanging leads to deformity of the CA arch, rotator cuff tears, subacromial impingement, the frozen shoulder and fraying or rupture of the bicep tendons. A common treatment for shoulder pain is cortisone injections. These injections should be avoided as they may make the problem worse by leading to infection, rotator cuff or biceps tendon ruptures, and nerve damage.

After rotator cuff repair surgery, it takes about six weeks for the tendons to heal initially; three months to form a relatively strong attachment to the bone and about six to nine months before the shoulder feels normal. The average time to return to unrestricted activity is 11 months. Physical therapy treatments will be necessary during the months of waiting for discharge from care. Failures are common. Judging from the results achieved by readers of this book, most have relieved their symptoms of the rotator cuff tear without the need for surgery.

The Frozen Shoulder
(Adhesive Capsulitis)

Inflammation of the shoulder lining may also cause shoulder stiffness resulting in a "frozen shoulder," or adhesive capsulitis. The cause is unknown. The exercises in the book will stretch the joint lining (the capsule) to relieve this condition.

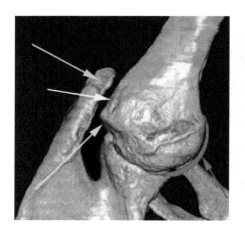 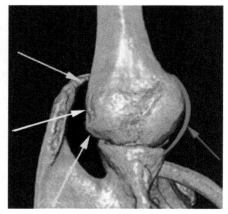

Fig. 57   **Fig. 58**

These two images show the stretching of the joint capsule (pink arcs, pink arrows) that takes place when one hangs. The image on the left shows the shortened capsule (pink arc). In the image on the right the capsule is lengthened by hanging (pink arc). Repeated hanging gradually stretches the shoulder joint capsule relieving the pain of the frozen shoulder and restoring motion. At the same time, while hanging, the humerus (yellow arrows) leans against the acromion (green arrows) bending this structure providing more room beneath the acromion. The aqua arrows indicate the site of attachment of the rotator cuff tendons. Pink arcs, artist's rendering.

The term "frozen shoulder" was first used by a Boston orthopedist, E.A. Codman. He stated in 1934 that the frozen shoulder was *"difficult to define, difficult to treat and difficult to explain."* More than 80 years later, we are still not much further. The frozen shoulder usually gets better without treatment after 12-18 months. Current treatment for the frozen shoulder includes 4-6 months physiotherapy, cortisone injections, manipulation under anesthesia and arthroscopic or open surgical release. Other treatments consist of acupuncture, massage, heat therapy, distension of the joint with anesthetic fluid and surgery. Complications from manipulation include fracture of the humerus, dislocation, and nerve injuries. The hanging exercise relieves nearly 95 % of cases in days, weeks, or months without pills, therapy or surgery.

Whether you have subacromial impingement, a rotator cuff tear or a frozen shoulder, the hanging exercise will not worsen the problem, and in most cases will return your shoulders to normal, pain-free function.

Some Suggestions for Hanging Equipment

Any number of free-standing hanging bars are available on the web. Hooked gloves and straps make the hanging exercise easier.

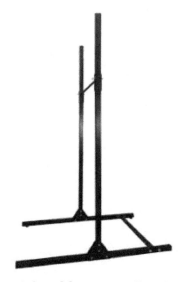

Fig. 59 One style of free-standing hanging bar.

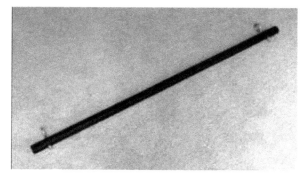

Fig. 60 This is a 1" diameter steel pipe with eye-bolts to be hung from the ceiling rafters or beams.

50

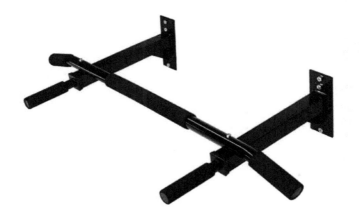

Fig. 61 A wall mounted chin-up bar. (Image from the web.)

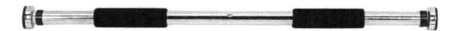

Fig. 62 Doorway hanging bar. (Image from the web.)

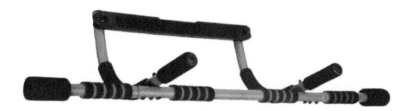

Fig. 63 An economical pull-up bar available at a number of stores. This bar is placed over a doorway casing and simply hangs without any fastening devices. It may not allow the full hanging exercise, but does allow partial hanging. Its simplicity makes it an excellent choice. (Image from the web.)

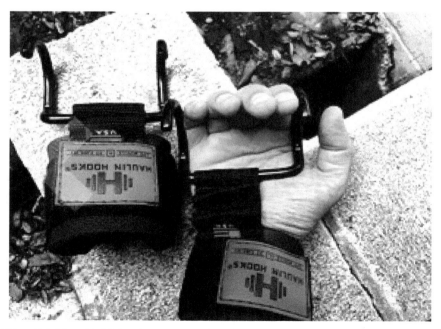

Fig. 64 Haulin' Hooks spare the fingers. Image from the web.

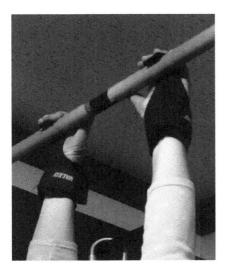
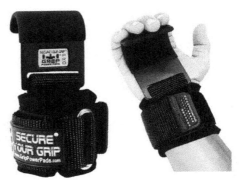

Fig. 65   **Fig. 66**

More wrist-based hanging hooks. Images from the web.

Making Your Own Hanging Bar

A free-standing hanging bar design.
A small stool may be used to reach the bar.

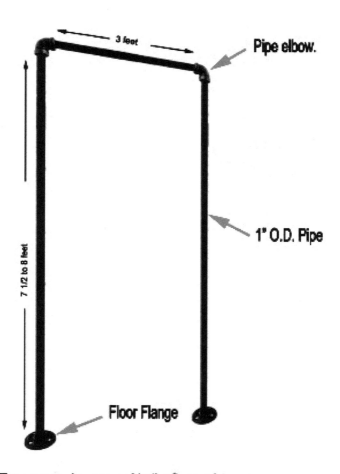

Flanges may be screwed to the floor or beams.

Fig. 67 An inexpensive free-standing bar may be built from simple, common pipe materials.

PART TWO
The Science

The remaining pages are devoted to further explanation of the science behind the exercise program. They present my theory as to why the hanging exercise restores the health of the shoulder and prevents further injury. They may also be of interest to therapists, surgeons and other healthcare workers. Some of the information and images are repeated for emphasis.

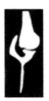

The Coracoacromial (CA) Arch

The CA arch is a curved structure in the shoulder that overlies the rotator cuff tendons and includes the acromion, the coracoacromial ligament and the coracoid process. An understanding of the CA arch is central to this book. This section of the book is devoted to helping you visualize what the CA arch is and why it may be stretched during the hanging exercise, and why this is of such importance. Because of the difficulty in presenting these 3D structures, it is hoped that viewing the shoulder from many perspectives may help overcome this difficulty. Viewing the volume (3D) images and videos at www.kirschshoulder.com or YouTube at "Dr. John Kirsch," from which many of the figures in this book are taken is recommended.

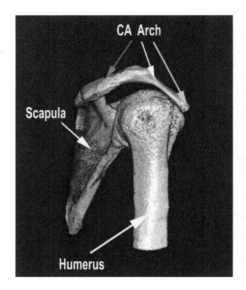
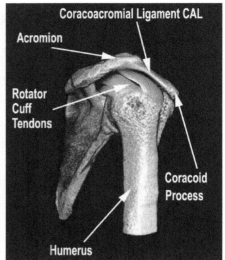

Fig. 68   **Fig. 69**

Fig. 68 is a CT scan with the subject holding the arm at the side. The CA arch consists of the acromion, red arrow; the coracoacromial ligament, white arrow; and the coracoid process, green arrow. **Fig. 69** The rotator cuff tendons have been added by the artist. It should be easy to understand from the position of the CA arch that it covers the structures beneath it, and if the compliance/flexibility of the arch is not maintained by repeated stretching by hanging, it may contract and press on the underlying rotator cuff causing impingement and tearing within the tendons. The CA arch has been stretched by hanging.

It is the contracture of the CA arch that is responsible for most of our troubles with our shoulders. It is the CA arch, if not stretched by overhead use of the arm including a hanging exercise that will contract, pressing on the rotator cuff causing irritation, inflammation, degeneration of the tendons and pain.

Beneath the CA arch is the space for the rotator cuff tendons that lift the arm and a thin sac of tissue called the subacromial bursa. If this space becomes too tight, the rotator cuff tendons moving beneath this CA arch will be pinched resulting in various degrees of pain and inflammation, degeneration and tearing of the tendons as well as some degree of irritation of the subacromial bursa. The bursa will be discussed later in the book.

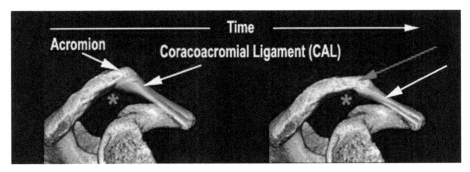

Fig. 70 An image showing how with ***time, gravity*** and ***disuse***; the acromion becomes hooked (red arrow) and the coracoacromial ligament (CAL) (white arrows) is contracted/ shortened, narrowing the space beneath the acromion. This narrowing causes pinching of the rotator cuff and the subacromial bursa, pain and eventually tears of the rotator cuff tendons. Pink asterisks, space for the rotator cuff and the subacromial bursa. Acromial bending: artist's rendering.

The daily life of modern man does not provide sufficient opportunity to properly stretch this important part of the shoulder, the CA arch. The hanging exercise, using the force of gravity, will provide the stretching that will reverse the process that led to the deformity. Hanging from an overhead support is an important normal human activity that modern man has neglected.

Another Joint in the Shoulder: The Acromiohumeral Joint

Never mentioned before, another articulation or joint in the shoulder was found doing the research for this book, the "acromiohumeral joint." It is a "part-time" joint that is a joint only when a person elevates the arm or hangs from an overhead support. If you search the web for "acromiohumeral," you will find that this term is applied only to an acromiohumeral *interval* with no mention of an acromiohumeral *joint*. I call the acromiohumeral joint a "joint" as there are few other terms that can be used to describe an articulation of one bone with another. When this joint is engaged by hanging, the upper humerus leans on the acromion exerting a bending force to the acromion.

It is this bending force applied to the acromion by the humerus that is nature's way of restoring and maintaining the health of the shoulder.

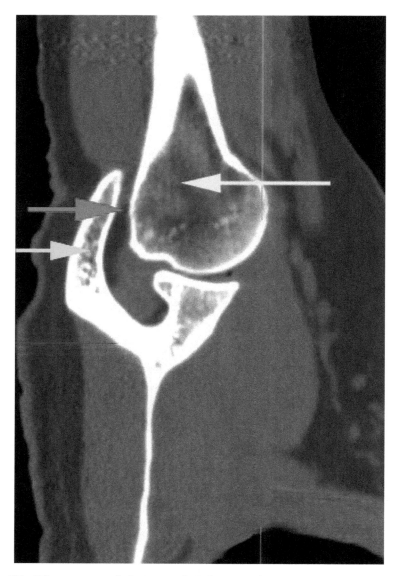

Fig. 71 The acromiohumeral joint: red arrow, the acromion: green arrow, the humerus: gold arrow. The joint is only visible while elevating the arm or hanging from a bar. The humerus leans on and bends the acromion.

Close-up View

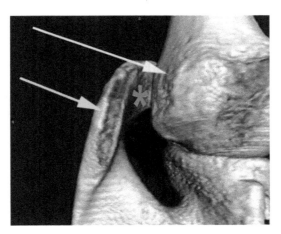

Fig. 72 A close-up view of the acromiohumeral joint (red asterisk) during simulated hanging. Yellow arrow, humerus.

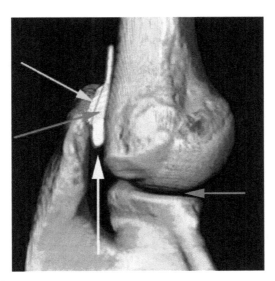

Fig. 73 Contents of the acromiohumeral joint (artist's rendering). The subacromial bursa: pink arrow, the coracoacromial ligament: aqua arrow, the glenohumeral joint; red arrow, the acromiohumeral joint space: white arrow.

The Acromiohumeral Joint: X-ray View

In order to view the acromiohumeral joint while raising the arm, a subject sat while the technician took an x-ray video of the subject raising and lowering the arm focusing on the space between the acromion and the humerus. The results of this effort are seen in the images below.

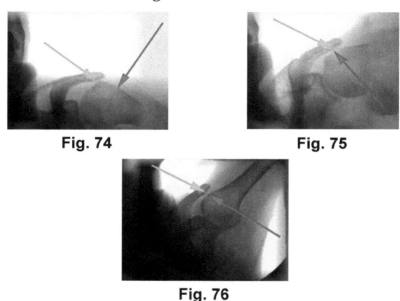

Fig. 74   **Fig. 75**

Fig. 76

As you can see in this series of images, the side of the humerus (red arrows) gradually moves to a position beneath the acromion to lean against the acromion (green arrows) gradually lifting and bending this structure. When you hang, this bending force is greatly increased and thereby *maintains* the space between these two structures preventing the subacromial impingement syndrome, rotator cuff tears and the frozen shoulder. In **Figs. 75 and 76**, the space between the arrows is the acromiohumeral joint. The video of these images can be viewed on the website: www.kirschshoulder.com or YouTube under "Dr. John Kirsch."

The acromiohumeral joint is a different kind of joint. There is no articular cartilage as in the synovial joints of the body — the hip, knee, shoulder glenohumeral joint, finger joints, ankle etc. The subacromial bursa and the coracoacromial ligament provide the lubrication and cushion necessary while hanging and elevating the arm. The joint is transitory and only present while elevating the arm or hanging from an overhead support.

The Two Main Joints in the Shoulder

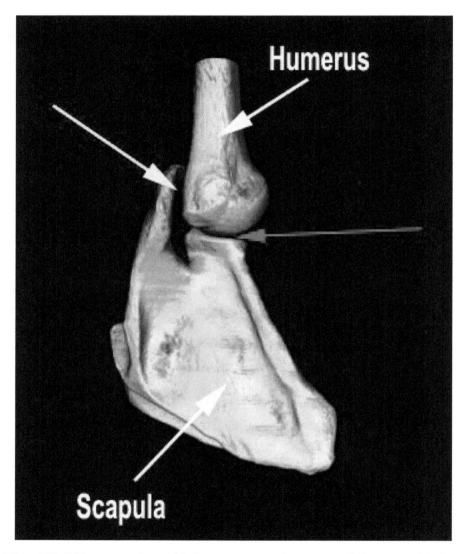

Fig. 77 CT scan view. Yellow arrow, the acromiohumeral joint; red arrow, the glenohumeral joint.

The Acromiohumeral Interval: X-ray View

Standard medical texts explain and discuss the acromiohumeral *interval*. There has never previously been mention of an acromiohumeral *joint*. Below are x-ray images of the acromiohumeral interval. This interval is the space between the acromion and the humeral head as seen on an x-ray as in the images on the next page.

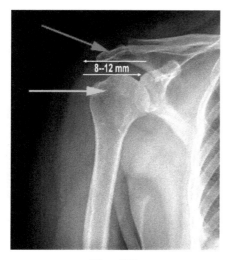 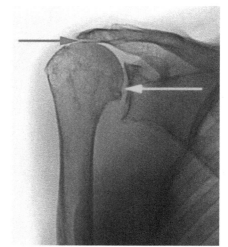

Fig. 78 **Fig. 79**

Fig. 78 Normal acromiohumeral interval. Red arrow, acromion; green arrow, humerus. The space between the white lines is the acromiohumeral interval. The normal interval distance is about 8-12 mm or 3/8." Normally, the rotator cuff occupies the acromiohumeral interval.

Fig. 79 When the rotator cuff Is torn, the humerus moves up narrowing the acromiohumeral interval (red arrow) distorting the glenohumeral (GH) joint (green arrow). This leads to osteoarthritis of the glenohumeral joint. Image adapted from the web.

CT Scan View of the Shoulder in a Simulated Hanging Position

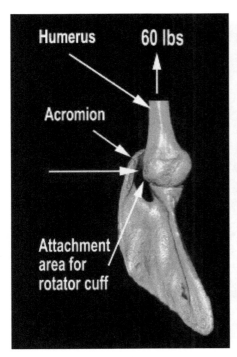
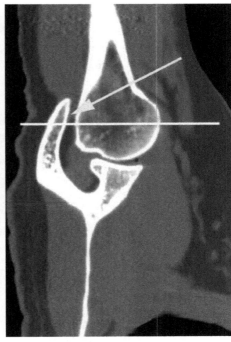

Humerus   60 lbs

Acromion

Attachment area for rotator cuff

Fig. 80   **Fig. 81**

Two CT scan side view images of the shoulder in the simulated hanging position with the subject holding a 60-pound weight. On the left Is the 3D skeletal image, on the right the CT scan sagittal, or "slice," image. Note how the humerus is positioned to lean on and exert a bending force to the acromion part of the CA arch. The axial image in **Fig. 83** below was taken from the level indicated by the horizontal white reference line in **Fig. 81** above. Yellow arrows, the acromiohumeral joint.

Slice or Axial Images

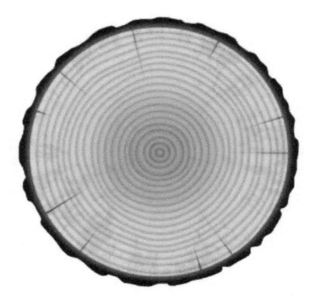

Fig. 82 Slice of a tree. Image adapted from the web.

The images on the next pages are "slice," or "axial," views of the shoulder from CT scans. Compare these to this slice of a tree.

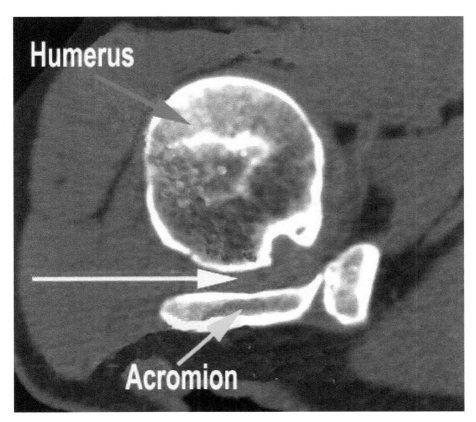

Fig. 83 This is an axial or 'slice' image made of the left shoulder in the hanging position seen from above. The level of this image is referenced in **Fig. 81** above by the horizontal white line. Notice the space (yellow arrow) between the humerus (blue arrow) and the acromion (green arrow). This space is occupied by the coracoacromial ligament (CAL) and parts of the bursal sac that eases the motion between the humerus and the CA arch. This space is the acromiohumeral joint (yellow arrow).

The Subacromial Bursa

As mentioned earlier in the book the bursa beneath the acromion would be discussed. The subacromial bursa is a thin-walled mostly empty pouch-like structure that helps the humerus and the overlying acromion glide smoothly when the arm is raised. In the image below, the bursa and the coracoacromial ligament (CAL) have been painted in by the artist to show their position.

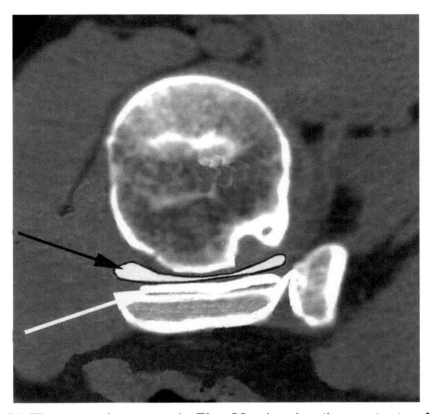

Fig. 84 The same image as in **Fig. 83,** showing the contents of the acromiohumeral joint with the subacromial bursa and the coracoacromial ligament tissue painted in by the artist. Black arrow, subacromial bursa; yellow arrow, coracoacromial ligament (CAL). The mostly empty bursa contains a small amount of serous fluid. The bursa and the ligament provide the lubrication for the acromiohumeral joint.

A note about these slice images of the shoulder taken in the hanging position at the level of the acromiohumeral joint. When you study these images picture yourself sitting and raising your left arm to full height or hanging from a bar. You will find then that your scapula with the acromion is behind your humerus and the humerus (upper arm) is in front of the acromion. You are looking down at a slice of your shoulder.

Subacromial Decompression Surgery

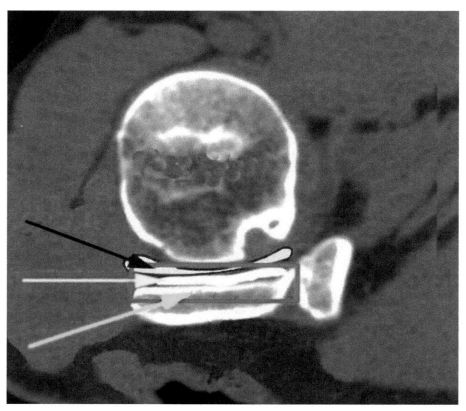

Fig. 85 The tissues inside the red rectangle are removed. Part of the subacromial bursa, black arrow; the coracoacromial ligament, yellow arrow and part of the acromion, green arrow are removed during subacromial decompression surgery (SAD). This surgery removes the most important parts of the acromiohumeral joint.

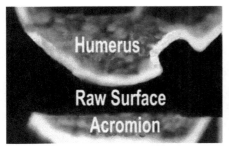

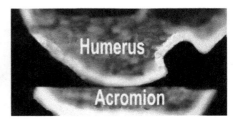

Fig. 86   **Fig. 87**

After subacromial decompression surgery (SAD), the acromion is left with a raw surface without the bursa or the coracoacromial ligament for lubrication. Then the acromion and the humerus migrate together causing painful grinding and failure of the subacromial decompression (SAD) surgery.

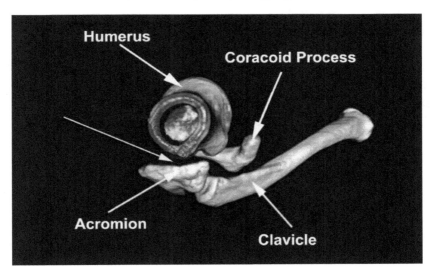

Fig. 88 The image shows the appearance of the left shoulder viewed from above in the hanging position with the subject facing forward. The image is taken from a CT scan study of a subject holding a 60-pound traction weight overhead to simulate the hanging position. Most of the humerus has been removed showing only the upper part of the humerus that presses on the acromion part of the CA arch. Notice where the humerus nearly touches the acromion. This space constitutes the acromiohumeral joint (yellow arrow).

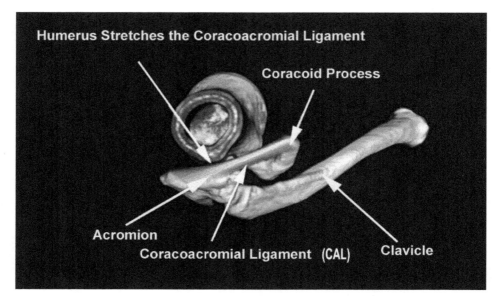

Humerus Stretches the Coracoacromial Ligament

Coracoid Process

Acromion

Coracoacromial Ligament (CAL)

Clavicle

Fig. 89 This is the same image as **Fig. 88.** with the coracoacromial (CAL) ligament part of the CA arch added by the artist. The CAL (ligament) connects the acromion and the coracoid process completing the CA arch. During the hanging exercise, this ligament is stretched along with the rest of the CA arch. The CAL has a broad insertion on the undersurface of the acromion that may well serve as a lubricating surface when the acromiohumeral joint is engaged with arm elevation or hanging. In fact, studies of the CAL tissue have found that the ligament inserting on the acromion has some of the properties of joint cartilage.

Shoulder CT Scan: Front View

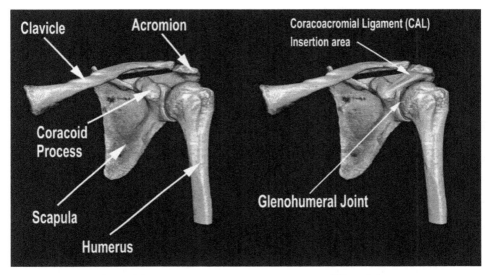

Fig. 90   **Fig. 91**

In **Fig. 91** the coracoacromial ligament (CAL) has been added by the artist. Note the insertion area for the ligament. The CAL has a broad insertion beneath the acromion. This allows the ligament to ease the motion of the humerus beneath the acromion.

Bending the Acromion by Hanging

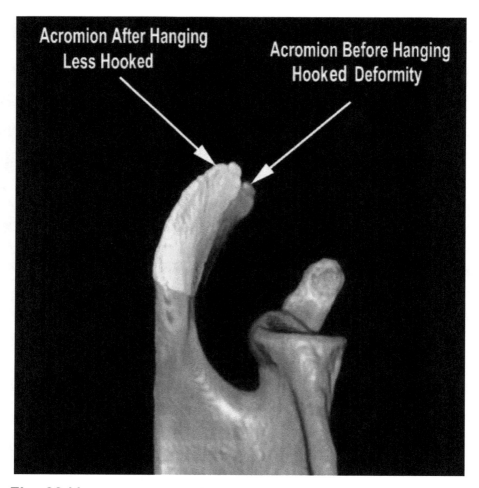

Fig. 92 You may correct the hooked deformity of the acromion by hanging. Author's conception (artist's rendering) of how the flexible acromion may be bent by the force of gravity to gradually remodel providing more room beneath the CA arch for the rotator cuff. The hooked deformity of the acromion is corrected (yellow acromion).

Arm Elevation Versus Hanging

Although full active arm elevation helps to lift the CA arch, more complete arm elevation is accomplished by hanging.

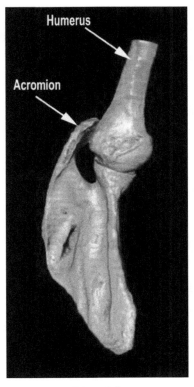

Fig. 93

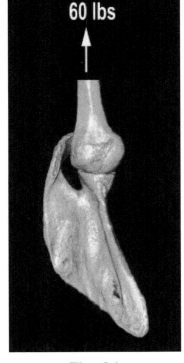

Fig. 94

3D CT images made with the subject in the CT scanner. The view is from the side of a right shoulder. On the left is an image with the subject in the scanner raising the arm with maximum effort. On the right is an image created with the subject holding a 60-pound weight to simulate hanging. Notice the more complete arm elevation in the image on the right. It is this stretching position while hanging that applies a reshaping or remodeling force to the acromion.

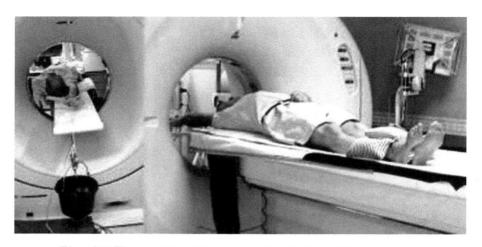

Fig. 95 The subject lying supine in the CT scanner.

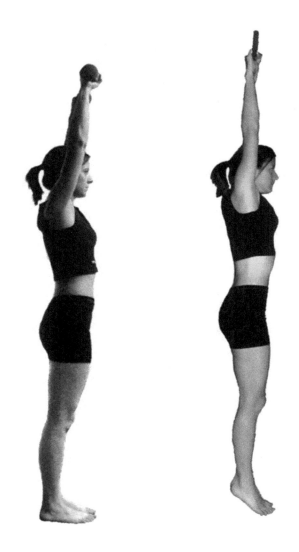

Fig. 96

Model demonstrating forward arm elevation versus hanging. Once again note the more complete arm elevation with hanging.

The Acromiohumeral Joint:
CT Scan Views While Hanging

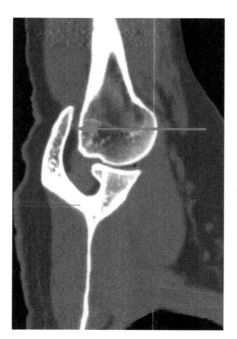 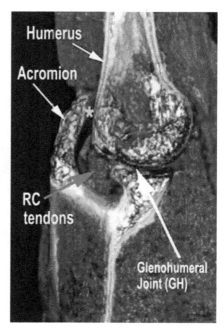

Fig. 97   **Fig. 98**

In **Fig. 97** red arrow, the acromiohumeral joint. In **Fig. 98** (soft tissue scan), note the safe position of the rotator cuff tendons (RC) and how the humerus bone leans on the acromion. The humerus pressing on the acromion gradually bends the acromion creating more room for the rotator cuff tendons (red arrow). The green asterisk indicates the acromiohumeral joint.

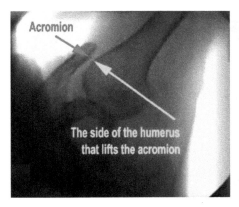

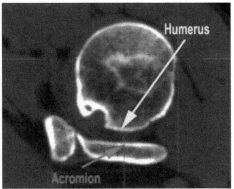

Fig. 99   **Fig. 100**

On the left, an x-ray video. CT scan axial/slice image on the right. The space between the arrows in both figures is the acromiohumeral joint.

Finding the CAL

Capturing an image of the coracoacromial ligament (CAL) with scanning equipment is exceedingly difficult. The ligament is quite thin, made of soft tissue and lies in an oblique plane. Most CT scan files saved in radiology facilities save only the vertical and horizontal "slice" images. However, using more powerful "Volume" or 3D digital imaging programs, it is possible to rotate and digitally dissect the skeleton and soft tissues finding the coracoacromial ligament in oblique views. If you search the web and textbooks you will not find any similar images of the ligament, making these images unique. The next two images exhibit the results of my search for the CAL.

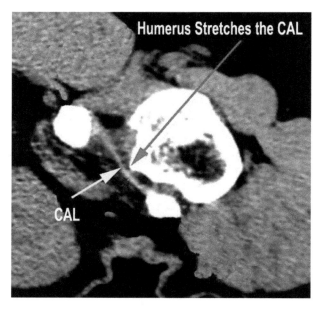

Fig. 101 This slice image was taken from a CT scan study of the subject's right shoulder in the simulated hanging position. The coracoacromial ligament (CAL) was found in its oblique plane along with the image of the humerus as it presses on and stretches the ligament during the hanging exercise.

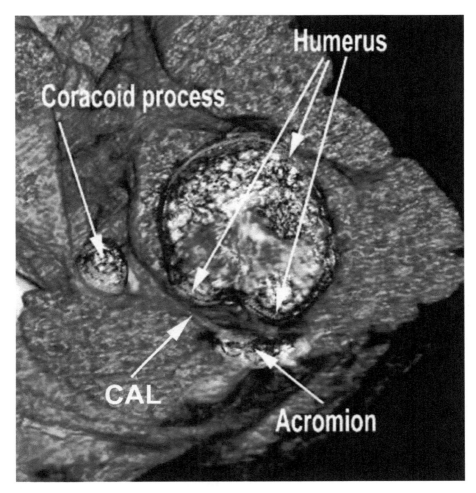

Fig. 102 This soft tissue slice image was created from a CT scan of a subject in the simulated hanging position. The CT editing program was set to show soft tissues (muscles, ligaments) and the volume image was cut in the plane of the coracoacromial ligament (the CAL). Note that the humerus while hanging is positioned to stretch the adjacent coracoacromial ligament (CAL) and bend the acromion. As the ligament part of the arch is soft tissue it is very difficult to capture with x-ray or CT scans. Yet with careful digital dissection of the CT scan image with a volume imaging editor, as you see here, it is possible.

85

The Humerus Bends the Acromion While Hanging

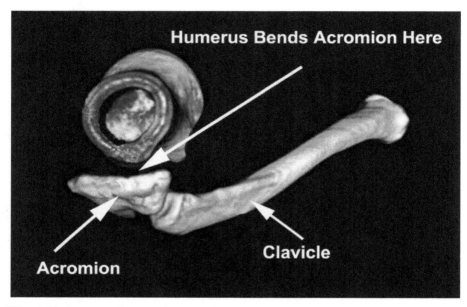

Fig.103 Image from above showing how the humerus leans on and bends the acromion while hanging. You will not immediately understand this image. You are looking down at your left shoulder from above while hanging. When you hang, your shoulder blade, the scapula with the acromion, is behind the humerus. It might even be more understandable if you think of being another person standing above you looking down at your skeleton.

The Human Pendulum

The slight oscillation or swinging that occurs when a person steps off a stool to reach and hang from an overhead bar might lend the idea that there could be over-rotation within the shoulder that could cause damage to the rotator cuff. Over-rotation could cause "internal impingement" of the rotator cuff. The only "joint" that can rotate when you hang is the top joint, the wrist. It is impossible for over-rotation or internal impingement to occur in the shoulder while hanging from an overhead support. This effect is seen in **Fig. 104**.

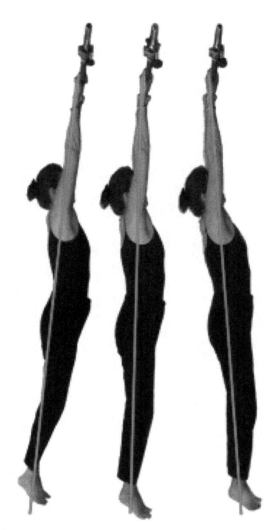

Fig. 104 The human pendulum. This image was composited from photos taken at separate moments during intentional exaggerated swinging of the subject as she performed the hanging exercise to demonstrate that the only joint that can rotate while hanging is the wrist. It is nearly impossible for over-rotation and internal impingement of the shoulder to occur while hanging from an over-head support.

Muscles Stretched While Hanging

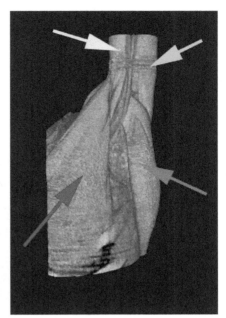

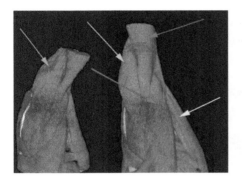

Fig. 105	Fig. 106

CT scan images captured with soft tissue setting. In **Fig. 105** while raising the arm and hanging. On the left, simple arm elevation, on the right, hanging. Elevation of the arm is much more complete while hanging. Green arrows, deltoid; blue arrow, latissimus dorsi; red arrow, triceps; yellow arrows, pectoral muscles. In **Fig. 106**, front view: blue arrow, pectoral muscles; yellow arrow, biceps; green arrow, triceps; red arrow, latissimus dorsi. Not only are the skeletal structures affected, but many muscles and other soft tissues are stretched. The hanging exercise and weight lifting return these muscles to a robust healthy condition.

Hanging for the Spine

Whenever you're upright, standing or sitting, gravity is tugging at your spine. Over time, gravity's power pulls your vertebrae down and compresses the discs. As a result, your height actually decreases as you age. Hanging from an overhead bar reverses the effects of gravity decompressing the spine and may over time prevent further destructive disc injury. It also strengthens the core back muscles. I suggest you hang from a bar daily, not only for your shoulders, but for your spine. Often, while hanging, you'll feel a "pop" in your spine. The tightness in your back is being relieved.

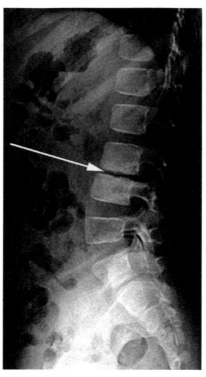

Fig. 107 Narrowed lumbar disc (white arrow). Image adapted from the web.

The Importance of Hanging Through the Ages

Briefly, the anthropologists who study the history of man are fairly certain that ancestral man was a creature that spent much of his time in the forest and would be considered arboreal, swinging and hanging from trees. Decreased overhead use of the arms may be related to the current epidemic of shoulder degenerative disease. Research shows that the incidence of shoulder problems, specifically rotator cuff disease is largely limited to man and rarely found in apes. This may be a result of man's abandoning brachiation. The evidence indicates that swinging, hanging and climbing remain important exercises for maintenance of the shoulder.

One of the important play activities for children in the U.S., the monkey bars have been declared too dangerous and have been phased out of most playgrounds and abandoned in physical education. Similarly, most modern physical training centers ignore swinging by the hands. This was a huge mistake; children loved the monkey bars for a reason. They were a playground feature important for the development of the upper body.

When a person hangs from an overhead support they are not only stretching the CA arch. There are many other ligaments, muscles and joints of the shoulder and between the shoulder and the thorax that by their very position in the human body must be stretched to their limit while hanging. Treat your shoulders and spine; go find a good tree to swing around on!

Again, video clips of the CT scans made during the research for this book showing the rotating shoulder in the hanging position, with and without muscles and ligaments, and other full color images taken from the CT scan studies are available at www.kirschshoulder.com or YouTube.

Therapists and physicians can provide many helpful treatments for your shoulders. But only you; doing the exercises presented in this book, can reshape and strengthen your own shoulders to recover and maintain painless normal shoulder activity. All people, both young and old, should do the exercises regularly to keep their shoulders healthy and prevent the deformities that lead to shoulder pain and injury. Hanging bars could be installed in many public places (airport lounges, bus stops) for all people to restore and maintain the health of their shoulders. Look around for an object to hang from: it won't be an easy search!

Man is a true brachiator. You must brachiate; or, at least simulate brachiation by frequent hanging from an overhead bar and lifting light weights to a full overhead position to maintain the health of your shoulders.

Again, the hanging exercise is not a panacea! The hanging exercise is not recommended for persons with unstable or dislocating shoulders, in precarious physical health, or with severe osteoporosis (fragile bones). If you have shoulder pain that goes unexplained for several weeks, it is wise to obtain a diagnosis from your physician.

Epilogue

Once again and finally we come to the articulation that over time has drawn little attention because it shows up only in certain positions (such as in hanging) and in certain radiographic images such as the CT scans in this book. It has never before been imaged. This is the acromiohumeral joint. While this has not been recognized historically as a "true" joint like the glenohumeral and the acromioclavicular joints, the hip and knee; its appearance during hanging establishes its existence, however transitory. This joint is as important as any other joint in the human body.

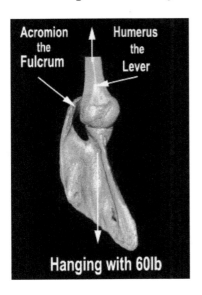

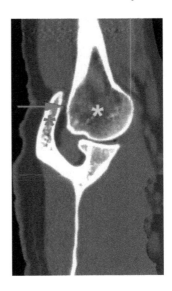

Fig. 108   **Fig. 109**

In **Fig. 108**, the shoulder skeleton seen while hanging. The humerus serves as a lever that leans on and bends the acromion, the fulcrum, maintaining the space between the humerus and acromion, and the weight of the body hanging produces maximal arm elevation. In **Fig. 109**, red arrow, the acromiohumeral joint; green asterisk, the humerus; and red asterisk, the acromion.

Over time, I have reached the conclusion that the acromiohumeral joint holds the key to the success of the hanging exercise. It was Archimedes who said "Give me a lever long enough and a fulcrum on which to place it, and I shall move the earth." The hanging program says "Give me a lever just the right size and I will pry the shoulder tissues back to normal." In hanging, the humerus becomes the lever, the acromion becomes the fulcrum, and the patient's weight provides the force to produce full arm elevation. **It is the acromiohumeral joint that maintains the health of the shoulder.**

Therapists have found that patients progress more rapidly when doing active exercises. In hanging, the patient controls his/her level of pain tolerance. Hanging provides just the right position of lever and fulcrum and the weight of the body is "QS" (Quantity Sufficient). The very best thing that can be said about the hanging exercise??? It's FREE!

And now I conclude with a final look at how the hanging exercise restores the shoulder without surgery.

Time

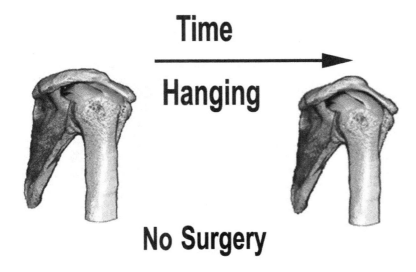

Hanging

No Surgery

Fig. 110 The hanging exercise, over time, restores the shoulder without pills, therapy or surgery. The acromion using **Wolff's Law** (pages 9 and 10) is gradually bent up to a normal configuration, and the coracoacromial ligament is stretched relieving the pressure and inflammation in the rotator cuff tendons.

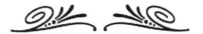

This then is the
Solution & Prevention
of most

Shoulder Pain Problems

Bibliography

1. Kottke, F.J., Pauley, D.L., Ptak, R.A., "The rationale for prolonged stretching for correction of shortening of connective tissue," *Arch Phys Med Rehabil.* 1966:47:347.0.

2. Wolff, Julius, *Das Gesetz der Transformation der Knochen,* August Hirschwald, Berlin, 1892.

3. Ziegler, D.W., Matsen, F.A. III, Harrington, R.M., "The superior rotator cuff tendon and acromion provide passive superior stability to the shoulder." Submitted to *J Bone Joint Surg.* 1996. P 32

9 781589 096424